Integration and Growth

Integration and Growth

Prof. Dr. Ceylan Das

Printed in the United States of America

Library of Congress Control Number: 2020924009
ISBN: Softcover   978-1-64908-632-7
              eBook   978-1-64908-631-0

Republished by: PageTurner Press and Media LLC
Publication Date: 01/15/2021

To order copies of this book, contact:
PageTurner Press and Media
Phone: 1-888-447-9651
order@pageturner.us
www.pageturner.us

CONTENTS

PART II: BASIC CONCEPTS

PART III: APPLICATION

To my children: Ceren and Buğra

PREFACE

Integration and growth. The magic strength of the Gestalt therapy approach is hidden in these two vast words. One of my clients beautifully expressed this in the following lines:

I wanted to grow, to be strong
I was so alone in this big world
Small and in pieces
Afraid of being alive And mostly of myself.

But I wanted to grow, to be strong
I first took a look at myself from a corner, hesitating
Then from another corner, shyly
The more I looked, the more I wanted to look
And I gathered whatever there is
I got rid of all that clutter
And I did put myself together, integrated.

I wanted to grow, to be strong
Then I looked at my loved ones
At the world which scared me
Looked at life and every living thing
The more I looked, the more I approached them
I saw them, they saw me
First we greeted each other, but it took a while
But then we hugged, oh so warmly

I gathered them and put them inside me

We are integrated

And suddenly I saw that what I wished for was now true

I had grown.

H. D.

This book is written with two important goals in mind. One of the aims of the book is to introduce the Gestalt therapy approach and, while introducing it, to help readers to understand themselves better. The second purpose of the book is to help those therapists in therapy training by presenting the theory and methods of the Gestalt approach with examples, and thus contribute to the raising of their therapeutic knowledge and skill levels. In order to achieve these goals, I put this book together by going over the literature of Fritz Perls, the founder of the Gestalt therapy approach, by reviewing the contributions of his followers and those of contemporary Gestalt therapists and adding my own views and experiences.

I organized and explained the information according to my own "gestalt," born from the training I have had over a long period at various Gestalt institutes in the USA and Europe. In other words, the theoretical and methodical information included in this book reflects how I understand the Gestalt approach and how I practice it. In almost all sections of the book, the information given is supported by examples from daily life, from my clients, and from technical practices. However, the Gestalt therapy approach has such a rich technical repertoire that it was not possible to cover it all in this book. Furthermore, a detailed investigation of all methods and techniques is not the purpose of this book. The examples given regarding therapeutic interventions are based on work I have carried out with my clients over the years. However, with due respect for confidentiality, which is of utmost importance in psychotherapy work, and in accord with ethical rules, all names and all identifying characteristics of the sample cases have been changed. On the other hand, as the Gestalt therapy approach is focused on what is experienced in the "here and now," it was rather difficult to fully convey in words what really was experienced during therapy and in particular the nonverbal and bodily reactions. Furthermore, since Gestalt therapy approach is based on a people-to-people dialogue, the written narrative of a dialogic relationship also emerged as another difficulty.

The book is divided into three parts. The first, the introduction, includes sections such as the development and fundamentals of the Gestalt theory approach, psychological health, therapeutic relations and the Gestalt therapist. The section on the development and fundamentals of the Gestalt therapy approach covers how it has integrated various opinions within itself and how it regards the human from existentialist, phenomenological, and holistic points of view. According to the Gestalt perspective, healthy people can take their own responsibilities, can actualize themselves, and are authentic and mature. Moving on from these characteristics, the ultimate goal of the therapy is to create people who are able to meet their own needs and who are in harmony with their environment without obstructing their growth and development. In the later part of the psychological health section, information is given on how the Gestalt approach can be used for almost all psychological problems that may come to mind, as well as for personal development within individual, couple, family, or group therapy. In the section on therapeutic relations and the Gestalt therapist, the importance of a dialogue relationship during therapy, that is, a deep person-to-person relationship, is emphasized. Within this relationship, the Gestalt therapist reflects his/her own personality, creativity, knowledge, and existence onto the therapy and works with and for the client without judging, interpreting, or labeling them.

In the second part of the book, the basic concepts of the Gestalt approach and how these are used in therapy are covered. The first concept given in this part is awareness, which is like an inland sea a person can reach for whenever in trouble and where he/she can access the source of those troubles. This can be very hard at times, but every voyage taken on this sea has a cooling and invigorating effect. The most important thing to be aware of during such a journey is one's needs. The more a person is aware of his/her needs, meets them as soon as possible and through the most appropriate means, the more he/she will feel happy, at peace, adequate, and safe. In the section entitled "Needs," the factors that prevent the satisfaction of needs and problems caused by the difficulties faced at different phases of the need-satisfaction cycle are discussed. One of the factors that prevent need satisfaction is unfinished business, which not only obstructs the meeting of a person's current and new needs, but also leads to a number of psychological problems due to the failure to satisfy past needs. Unfinished business that is related to deep unmet needs causes the formation of fixed gestalts and affects the current existence of the person not only emotionally and mentally but also physically.

Another significant concept in terms of the Gestalt approach is contact. Its importance comes from the belief that a person can only integrate and grow through contact, by meeting him/herself and the environment. The most important barriers that prevent the integration and growth of the person are the contact styles used in this meeting. Each of the styles of contact, which are called in the Gestalt approach introjection, desensitization, deflection, projection, retroflection, egotism, and confluence, is taken up in detail in separate sections, which cover the definition, the advantages and disadvantages, the basis of each contact style as well as the personality characteristics of people who use them frequently and how to work with them in therapy. Introjection, which forms the basis of the other styles of contact, is a way of contact that depends on the messages a person has taken from the environment while growing up, that is, on what information he/she has introjected. Introjects determine how the person regards the world and him/herself. Desensitization, which is generally developed to enable the person to cope with highly traumatic experiences, leads to numbness in a person, preventing him/her from enjoying life, being happy and joyful. The next style of contact, deflection, by causing a person to reject positive or negative external reactions, while protecting him/her against negative reactions, also prevents that person from hearing and assimilating the positive ones. Projection means attributing the person's unique characteristics, thoughts and feelings, whether or not he/she is aware of them, onto his/her environment. How we perceive the people and the environment around us is defined by our projections. In this sense, the people and the world around us are a projection screen that we have created according to our perceptions. A person who uses retroflection as a style of contact does not go to the environment to meet his/her needs and appears to have condemned him/herself to meeting his/her needs on his/her own. While this in a way makes the person feel strong, when used chronically, it could make him/her feel lonely and eventually psychologically weakened as contact with the environment is blocked. In the style of contact known as egotism, instead of living his/her life as if watching a film based on his/her life where he/she has the leading role, a person focuses solely on the leading actor—him/herself. Hence, people who use egotism frequently can find it very hard to go beyond themselves and contact others. People who try to contact through confluence do not behave like themselves. Since they greatly fear being alone, criticized, or excluded, they cannot put forward their own wishes and ideas, cannot say no to anybody, and do not own their needs. Since they lack the power for self-support, they continuously need the approval and support of others.

Integration of polarities is one of the primary goals of the Gestalt approach. In the section on polarities, it is mentioned that personality traits are located on a dimension with opposite traits at the different ends. The evaluation of these polarities, or personality traits, as positive or negative is not determined according to the values of society but according to the needs of the person and his/her environmental conditions. For this reason, the person has to claim the personality characteristics at both poles. Disclaimed poles lead to the emergence of inner conflicts that lead to neurotic symptoms.

The third part of the book emphasizes what should be taken into consideration in understanding humans and their integration and growth according to the Gestalt approach. In this part, which includes practice-oriented information, firstly the concept of resistance that obstructs growth and development is discussed. According to the Gestalt approach, resistance is not a situation that should be hastily and forcefully eliminated during therapy. On the contrary, it is a case that should be understood, investigated, and experienced. In the Gestalt approach, in order for the clients to be ready for growth and integration, they first of all need a therapist who accepts them as they are, including their resistances, and who respects them. Work on bodily reactions, physical complaints, body structure and posture—in short, work on body language—is very useful in recognizing impasses, unfinished business, creative adjustment, dysfunctional contact styles and polarities as well as resistances. The section on body language gives examples of methods that may be used during therapy and shows how integration of body, mind, and soul can be achieved.

According to the Gestalt approach, one of the paths to integration is dreams. Dreamwork is very important in therapy since dreams serve a purpose in the recognition of the rejected and disowned parts of the personality and their integration, the recognition of needs and the determination of existential messages, and the recognition and changing of unhealthy styles of contact in interpersonal relations. Hence, Gestalt therapy offers a wealth of methods for working with dreams. In a case presentation, which is the last subsection of the book, which maps could be used while diagnosing according to the Gestalt approach, the points that should be taken into consideration during therapy and the therapy process are explained through a real-life case.

The Gestalt therapy approach enables the achievement of highly impressive results in cases of numerous psychological problems. In the achievement of these successful results, the role of the various and creative methods it offers is significant. However, it should never be forgotten that the success of the Gestalt therapy approach is not merely dependent on the methods it offers. For the therapy to be successful, the therapist must have integrated the points of view and theoretical bases of the Gestalt approach into him/herself. Therefore, unless the reader has completed Gestalt therapy training, gone through therapy him/herself and had supervision for a sufficient period from a qualified Gestalt therapist, practicing these methods would be both extremely harmful and unethical.

Lastly, I hope that this book can contribute to your being more aware of yourself and those around you, to your integration with yourself and the world without judging or accusing, without feeling ashamed, scared or worried, and to exist as fully-grown and as you are.

ACKNOWLEDGMENTS

I first of all like to extend my sincere gratitude to my teachers at the Gestalt Therapy Center and Metanoia Institute in England, where I started my training, Petruska Clarkson, Talie-Levine Bar, Lynda Osborn, Sue Fisher, and my supervisors Todd Buttler and Marianne Fry, who supported and helped me in learning all the information and methods included in this book, integrating them and using them according to my personality, my past, and my culture. I would also like to thank my trainers at the Los Angeles Gestalt Therapy Institute during the later years of my training Robert and Rita Resnick, Todd Burley and Vernon de Riet. I am grateful for the support and help they gave at the last stage of my training, to Judith Hemming from the Systematic Training Center in England and to Anne Teachworth from New Orleans Therapy Institute in working with couples in therapy, to Ruella Frank in working with the body and to Ansel Wolt who generously helped in the work on Scale of Contact Styles mentioned in the book. Furthermore, my eternal thanks to my teacher and supervisor Paul Rebelliot, who is the founder of the San Francisco Gestalt and Existential Training School in whose work I participated with great admiration and who permitted me to practice the techniques he developed in Turkey and who supported me in developing my own.

I would like to thank from the depths of my heart and with all my sincerity to my clients who gave me the opportunity of practicing the knowledge and techniques I learned, who allowed me to be with them in their difficult moments, who put themselves forward as they were and who accepted me as I am, and to my students for encouraging me to write this book.

My thanks also go to my dear daughter Ceren and my son Buğra for the patience and understanding they showed during my studies. I am also really thankful to Aydan Erim who showed great care and attention in the translation of this book, to Robert West for his attentive efforts for the proofreading, and to Gözde Akkın for her creative designs and images.

PART I:
INTRODUCTION

1

DEVELOPMENT AND FUNDAMENTALS OF THE GESTALT THERAPY APPROACH

Fritz (Frederick) Perls, Laura Perls, and Paul Goodman started to develop the Gestalt therapy approach in the 1940s. At the very start, some ambiguity was experienced concerning the title of this therapy approach. In his first book entitled *Ego, Hunger and Aggression*, Fritz Perls (1947/1992, 219) gave it the title of "concentration" therapy, due to its especial focus on the "process" and "awareness." Another suitable name suggested for this therapy approach was "existential therapy" (Korb, Gorrell, and Van de Riet 1989, 1). However, toward the end of the 1940s, Fritz and Laura Perls attended a meeting held in New York along with other therapists who were working on this therapy approach at the time and decided on the name "Gestalt therapy approach." The influence of the perception studies conducted by Gestalt psychologists such as Wertheimer, Koffka, and Kohler and the holistic point of view of this approach were significant in the selection of the name (Estrup 2000). During this period, there were some who argued that the use of this name wasn't completely appropriate, as Gestalt therapy approach and Gestalt psychology are two different disciplines. Despite such arguments, Fritz Perls did not forego this name, and later Yontef (1982) demonstrated that in terms of its philosophy, the fundamentalmethods of Gestalt therapy are based on the information collected from Gestalt psychology, and Wheeler (1998, 12–41) thoroughly examined the histories of Gestalt psychology and Gestalt therapy. The role of the perception studies of Gestalt psychologists on Gestalt psychotherapy theory will be given in more detail later in this chapter.

Gestalt is a German word and has no entirely accurate correspondence in English. For this reason, it is not possible to describe its meaning with a single word. Thus, *Gestalt* is a word for a complete pattern or configuration (Korb et al. 1989, 1). It represents a unified whole that cannot be broken without destroying its nature. In order to define *Gestalt*, three phenomena should be mentioned. The first of these is a thing (or person, animal, color or anything), the second is the context or environment in which this object is located, and the third is the relation between them.

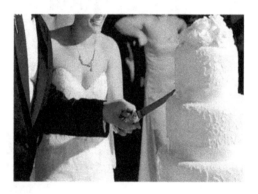

The bride and groom cutting the wedding cake

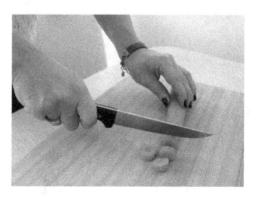

A woman cutting the carrot

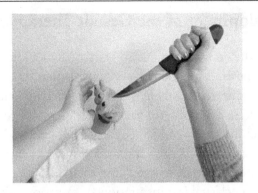

A woman stabbing a person

For example, as seen above, there are three different illustrations that include the same knife. Despite the presence of the same knife in each illustration, each constitutes a different gestalt, and the emotions, thoughts, and associations evoked by these different gestalts are consequently different. In other words, the knife in each illustration has a different meaning depending on its context and thus constitutes a different gestalt.

Just a short time after the publication of the book entitled *Gestalt Therapy: Excitement and Growth in Human Psychology* written jointly by Perls, Hefferline, and Goodman (1951), Fritz and Laura established the first Gestalt institute in New York. The second institute was established in Cleveland under the guidance of Fritz and Laura, and with contributions from Paul Goodman and Isodore From. The Gestalt therapy approach started to become popular in the 1960s with the studies of Perls in the Esalen Institute, California. Today, there are more than four hundred Gestalt institutes in the United States. Additionally, there are numerous Gestalt institutes or centers that provide therapy training in various countries of Europe, Asia, and even Australia. This approach is used in many parts of the world, and various meetings, conferences, and congresses are held on Gestalt therapy. In addition to that, there are Gestalt journals in Russian, French, German, Spanish, Norwegian, Portuguese, and Turkish as well as in English.

3

The Development of the Gestalt Therapy Approach

One of the most significant statements of field theory that constitutes the basis of the Gestalt approach is that "the whole is always more than and different from the sum of its parts." Parallel to that, the Gestalt approach has integrated a variety of therapy approaches, theories, and perspectives into itself and has consequently emerged as a "more and different" approach. Fritz Perls's acknowledgement of exciting ideas of his time and his intelligence in reorganizing these ideas were significant for the Gestalt approach's taking inspiration from various opinions (Estrup 2000). Below, you may find how and by which ideas Perls was inspired when creating the Gestalt therapy approach. These are summarized using Perls (1969/1992), Clarkson and Mackewn (1993, 1–29), and Estrup (2000) as references.

Perls was born in Berlin on July 8, 1893, to a Jewish family as the third and youngest child. His childhood and youth passed in an environment where significant developments took place in fields of science such as physics, chemistry, physiology, as well as literature and peace. Perls began his university education in the Faculty of Medicine of Berlin University and joined the army upon the start of World War I. After the war, Perls continued his education and graduated as a neuropsychiatrist. During this period, Perls's interest in the arts increased, and he met a variety of writers, poets, actors, actresses, dancers, and architects. These meetings led Perls to think that art, dance, and movement can be spontaneous and creative ways to express oneself, and later, he utilized them in his Gestalt therapy practices. In the meantime, Perls came across philosopher Sigmund Friedlander. Greatly impressed by his idea that "opposites define each other and opposites have a resting point in the middle," Perls integrated this idea into his theory in the following years.

Perls began his training in psychoanalysis with the effect of his first analyst, Karen Horney. Horney's opinions on therapeutic relations also had an impact on Perls's approach to dialogue. In the same period, Perls attended courses on Gestalt psychology. Thence, he deepened this knowledge of perception in the light of the studies of Gestalt psychologists such as Wertheimer, Koffka, and Köhler, and later, he utilized a set of main principles that stemmed from perception studies while developing his approach. One of the principles that Perls took into consideration was "people merely perceive things that draw their attention and by giving a meaning to those things within a whole, they form a gestalt or a figure." Perls was also influenced by Zeigarnik's (1927) statement that "people tend to remember the tasks they have not completed rather than the ones they have" and Ovsiankina's (1928) statement that "people have a tendency to complete unfinished tasks and make meaning out of incomplete information." In that period, Perls met Goldstein, who was deeply interested in Gestalt psychology and ran studies on brain-injured soldiers. Being an academician, Goldstein (1939) discovered during his researches that any damaged part of the body affects the whole organism and that the organism as a whole is attempting to repair this damage; in other words, the organism as a whole is in search of actualizing itself. Perls, deeply inspired by the studies of Goldstein, adopted Goldstein's opinions regarding "self- actualization," "functioning of the organism as a whole," and "all parts of the organism being in relation to each other" in the development of his own theory.

While attending courses on Gestalt psychology, Perls met Lore Posner, who would be known as Laura Perls and would later be his wife. In those days, Lore was interested in existentialism and phenomenological methods and was working with existentialists such as Buber and Tillich and with Husserl, who was a phenomenologist. Later, Lore's studies on existentialism and phenomenology had a considerable impact upon the future development of Gestalt therapy. Perls was also impressed by the existentialist perspective and introduced the concepts of freedom, responsibility, authenticity, and anxiety to Gestalt therapy. Furthermore, he incorporated both existentialist and phenomenological perspectives and gave a place to ideas that "people have a tendency to give meaning to their lives," that "there is no single indisputable truth," and "truth may differ from person to person and from one perspective to another" in his approach.

Meanwhile, Perls completed his Freudian psychoanalysis training and got his degree. Although he believed that much of the philosophy and methods of psychoanalysis were ancient, he attached great importance to Freud's opinions. Afterward, although he criticized, altered, and rejected some of Freud's ideas, he used several of Freud's opinions such as "the organism, the living things are in search of a homeostatic balance," "neurosis and psychosis have a meaning for that person," "childhood has an influence upon adulthood behavior" while developing Gestalt therapy approach. Affected by the significance Freud gave to dreams, Perls added dreamwork to the Gestalt therapy approach, but his way of working with dreams was totally different than Freud's. Perls was not only influenced by Freud but by many psychoanalysts, especially those who rejected orthodox psychoanalytical approaches. For example, he integrated into Gestalt practices the "active techniques" of Ferenczi, the "creative imagination techniques" of Jung, and the "here and now" approach used by Otto Rank in dream studies.

All the way along, because of his training, Perls worked with a number of therapists and supervisors. One of them was Eugene Harnik. Believing in passive analysis, Harnik remained silent during much of their sessions. After one and a half years, Perls quit therapy, and soon after, he learned that his therapist had been diagnosed with paranoia. This negative experience had a tremendously adverse effect on Perl's professional and philosophical development, which led him to question many aspects of psychoanalysis, especially those aspects of the analysis with Harnik, which he found very disturbing. He ended up with the opinion that in Gestalt therapy, the therapist–client relationship must be different to the relation in analysis and emphasized the importance of contact between the therapist and client. According to Perls, contact must be experienced fully in the therapy session and in the therapy room, or in other words, contact must be experienced in the "here and now." He also added that for good contact instead of "interpreting," phenomenological perspective must be used.

Following the disappointing experience with his former therapist, Perls began searching for a new therapist and, with the suggestion of his first therapist Horney, started working with Wilhelm Reich. Although Reich was a psychoanalyst, he was a critic of psychoanalysis, and he suggested that people store both emotional memories and the defenses against those memories in the form of muscular contractions and body armour. Perls, being greatly impressed with Reich's ideas related to the body, decided to integrate his suggestions in his own therapy approach. Laura and Fritz got married in 1929. In 1933, as Germany's Nazi Party acquired more power and Hitler initiated genocide against the Jewish population, Perls was forced to seek refuge in Holland. Later, he and his family put down roots in South Africa where he and his wife established the first institute for psychoanalysis. In South Africa, Perls path crossed with Smutz who was the prime minister, an accomplished general and philosopher of that time, and was deeply impressed by his book *Holism and Evolution*. Moving on from the rules of physics, the book also encompassed Gestalt psychology and field theory and suggested that "everything has a field" and "things and organisms are unintelligible if considered without these fields." Perls, focusing on ideas in the book such as "all things are in an incessant process of creative change" and "every living thing functions according to its structure and in a holistic way," integrated them into his therapy approach.

Perls later took part in World War II, and following the war, he and his family moved to New York from South Africa. Subsequently, in New York, Fritz and Laura Perls started to run weekly training/therapy sessions on the therapy approach they had been developing and exchanged ideas with various therapists participating in the groups. During these sessions, Perls met Sullivan and highly appreciated his "interpersonal psychoanalysis" movement. Sullivan's ideas such as "mental illnesses is a reaction to the events taking place between the person and his environment" and "the most important factor for a successful therapy is the relationship between the therapist and the patient" played a significant role in Perls's focusing on "here and now" and addressing the relationship between the person and his environment as a whole. Weisz, whom he met during group sessions, was another important name for Perls. With Weisz's influence, Perls started to gain interest in Zen Buddhism and realized remarkable similarities between his own opinions and those of Zen Buddhism. For instance, Perls' "here and now awareness" and the notion of "mindfulness" in Zen Buddhism or his "paradoxical theory of change" and the notion of "paradox" in Zen Buddhism had much in common. Perls was also affected by Moreno, the founder of the psychodrama approach, who integrated psychology and drama and stressed the significance of "encounter." Impressed by techniques of psychodrama such as "empty chair" and "hot seat," Perls incorporated them into his own therapy practice, but in the Gestalt approach, these techniques are used in a different way than they are in psychodrama.

Consequently, Fritz Perls harmonized all the mentioned viewpointswithin his own approach and, together with Laura Perls and Paul Goodman, developed the Gestalt therapy approach. He continued to run workshops and training sessions in Vancouver Island, Canada, during the last years of his life and passed away on March 14, 1970, after a battle with pancreatic cancer.

As can be understood, the Gestalt therapy approach, starting with psychoanalysis, was influenced by various theories and viewpoints and was eventually structured on existentialist, holistic, and phenomenological bases. In order to be able to understand Gestalt therapy better, these three perspectives will be given in detail below.

Fundamentals of the Gestalt Therapy Approach

Existentialist Perspective

Laura Perls had an immense impact on the existentialist foundations of the Gestalt approach. The existentialist perspective can be summarized through the concepts of the life-death dilemma, the meaning of life, anxiety, and responsibility. All living things are born with two innate goals: the first is survival; and the second is growth (Perls 1973, 7). Each plant, animal, or human being is able to survive, grow, and develop when the appropriate conditions are met. Nonetheless, unlike other living beings, it is not predetermined in which direction human beings will grow. According to the existentialist perspective, life does not have a predetermined meaning. Individuals themselves have to give a meaning to their lives. In other words, one must take responsibility for one's own existence (Smith 1977, 15) and decide in which direction he/she will develop and grow. Along with the responsibility of determining the meaning of their lives, individuals are also responsible for their feelings, the meanings they attribute to their experiences, and the ways they choose to cope with these experiences. Even though people do not have the freedom to choose their parents, the environment into which they are born, or the culture and conditions in which they grow up, they do have the freedom to choose what to accept or reject, how to think, how to feel, and what to do (Estrup 2000). Therefore, the existentialist perspective states that people are always capable of choosing and re-creating themselves.

According to the existentialist perspective all living things have the drive to actualize themselves, that is, "to be as they are" and "to reveal their existent potentials, characteristics and sides." However, social values and prohibitions lead the person to deny, suppress, or be ashamed of his/her innate and idiosyncratic aspects (such as sexuality, anger, crying, etc.). This causes the individual to be alienated from him/herself and leads the individual not to him/herself but to his/her self-image. Thus the individual will end up not actualizing him/herself but his/her self-image (Perls 1973, 99). Among all living things, only human beings strive to "become" something "they are not," which is actually contradictory with raison d'être. The existentialist perspective suggests that all we need is to accept who we really are and face up to life and the situations around us authentically (Clarkson and Mackewn 1993, 38).

During self-actualization, people rediscover themselves continuously, or in other words, they become aware of their needs, their feelings, and their thoughts and they reshape their lives accordingly. As personal needs, feelings, and thoughts are ever changing through the course of life, new problems, new opportunities, and new alternatives always emerge (Simkin and Yontef, 1984, 280). On the other hand, people are also aware of the fact they will one day perish. Searching for the meaning of life, on the one hand, and existential facts such as death, aloneness, isolation, uncertainty, freedom, and responsibility on the other, leads to anxiety. Existential anxiety is a normal state of being, and this anxiety leads us to new goals, new choices, and to live "fully" (Joyce and Sills 2003, 37). It is important to differentiate between existential anxiety and neurotic anxiety. Unlike existential anxiety, neurotic anxiety prevents the individual from living in the "here and now" and "as it is."

According to Perls (1973, 50), awareness of and responsibility for the total field, for the self as well as the other, give meaning and pattern to the individual's life. While trying to give a meaning to one's life, if a person avoids the existential facts such as death, aloneness, and ambiguity, instead of accepting and living with them, fixed gestalts are

9

formed. For instance, a child who lost his/her mother may decide "not to feel close to anyone and not to love anyone too much" and to stay away from people throughout all his/her life in order to avoid the fear of loss and pain again, or a woman who does not want to face the fact of aging and death may opt to receive numerous reconstructive surgeries. Another one by denying the fact that everybody is unique and alone may always seek another's company and avoid staying alone at all costs. Fixed gestalts such as avoiding people, frequent plastic surgeries, and always seeking another's company would block self-actualization.

Phenomenological Perspective

In the broadest sense, phenomenology is the individual's perception and understanding of him/herself and his/her environment in his/her unique way (Estrup 2000). According to the phenomenological perspective, the generally accepted meaning of an event, a situation, an object, etc., is not important. What is important is the specific and subjective meaning of those in that specific time and field for the person (Mackewn 1999, 58). Perls (1947/1992, 35) elaborates the concept of phenomenology through the example of a cornfield. Objectively, a cornfield is where planted corn seeds grow. But, apart from its objective meaning, this cornfield may have different and subjective meanings for different people depending on their own specific needs and situations. For example, a cornfield may have the meaning of sustaining livelihood for a farmer, a field for a forced landing for a pilot, a nice view to reflect on canvas for a painter, or a place far from prying eyes for two lovers to be alone. An individual's phenomenology is not only determined by "how" the individual perceives and attaches meaning to the environment but also "what" the individual perceives and attaches meaning to, or in other words, what he/she is aware of. To have a better understanding, look at the photograph below and determine the first three features that initially draw your attention. If possible, show the photograph to a friend or someone nearby and ask them to name the first three significant features that draw his/her attention. Most probably, the features that draw your and the other person's attention, the sequence of these features, and the reasons for their drawing your attention will be different, depending on your own phenomenology.

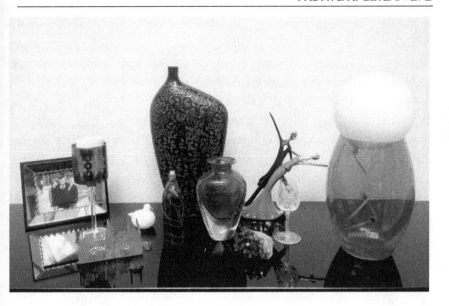

In summary, according to the phenomenological perspective, the meaning of everything is specific to that person and to that particular moment. Therefore, with respect to its phenomenological basis, there is no room for interpretations and generalizations in the Gestalt therapy approach as they are based not on specific personal meanings but on general assumptions. In other words, interpretations and generalizations are based on generally accepted truths and beliefs. For instance, some therapy approaches assume crossing one's arms to be an indication of "not being open to communication," whereas there might be a number of personal reasons for that persons' crossing his arms in that particular moment such as feeling cold, angry, ashamed, lonely, or just assuming that posture as a habit. In fact, only that person can know the meaning of his crossing his arms, therefore the therapist's interpretations of his posture may be meaningless or totally wrong. Perls considered the Gestalt approach as the only therapy approach that is based entirely on phenomenological principles. Yontef (1979) has also defined Gestalt therapy as clinical phenomenology.

Holistic Perspective

The holistic perspective is the most distinctive feature of the Gestalt therapy approach compared to other therapy approaches. According to the holistic perspective, the whole is formed by its constituent parts functioning together and in a collaborative way. Therefore, the whole cannot be explained by addressing its constituent parts or features individually. In order to explain this, Huckabay (1992, 306) used a metaphor regarding the descriptions made by three blind men of an elephant. The three blind men were brought next to an elephant, and they were requested to touch it and then to describe what they had just touched. The man who touched the tusk described the elephant as smooth and hard, the man who touched the tail described it as long and round, like a snake or a garden hose, and the man who touched the flank described it as baggy, bumpy, and hairy. Obviously all the definitions reflect a different feature of an elephant; however, none of them provides a definition of the elephant as a whole.

Likewise, it is not possible to define a person with regard to some of his characteristics only. The ability to understand a person can only be achieved by "seeing" him as a whole. This is why the Gestalt approach handles the person as a whole with his/her feelings, thoughts, and body. In other words, according to the holistic perspective, the body, the mind, and the soul are different aspects of the same thing (Perls 1947/1992, 21). Therefore, in terms of human health, the differentiation of mental-physical or bodily-spiritual is highly artificial. Bodily, emotional, and mental experiences cannot be separated from each other, and a change occurring in any one of them would affect the others, resulting in an effect on the organism as a whole. Perls (1973, 53) mentioned that, concentrating on the mental-physical or mind-body split preserves neurosis instead of curing it.

Just as it is not possible to evaluate physical and mental or bodily and spiritual separately, it is not possible to evaluate the two hemispheres of the brain separately either. The brain consists of two hemispheres, left and right. The left hemisphere is related to rational thoughts, causal explanations, and deductive postulates, and the right hemisphere is related to rhythms, spatial relations, and intuitions (Ornstein 1972). The Gestalt therapy approach tries to understand the person with all the characteristics of the two hemispheres that is with his/her sensations, perceptions, emotions, and thoughts as a whole. Perls (1948) criticizes psychoanalytical and behavioral therapy approaches for focusing merely on logic, causality, and analysis, or in other words, for paying attention only to the left hemisphere. Perls believed that the overvaluing of these rational, causal activities had created a split between deliberate behavior and spontaneous being, a split that was the cause of much malaise both in the individual and in society (Clarkson and Mackewn 1993, 36). On these grounds, in the Gestalt approach, the client is encouraged not only to express oneself with his/her thoughts but with his/her body, voice, artistic creations as well as with his/her feelings.

With the influence of the holistic perspective, in Gestalt therapy, the person is not only treated as a whole in him/herself but also as a whole with his or her environment. The Gestalt approach suggests that a person is both an individual and a social being; hence the person and the society are in constant interaction. In other words, the individual and his/her environment are a mutual interdependent, integrated system, where any change in one will affect the other (Perls 1973, 17). In terms of psychological health, it is wrong to examine the person or the society separately or to hold responsible either party for the emerging problems. That is to say that, in the emergence of psychological problems, the contact between the person and his/her environment is important.

Consequently, the Gestalt therapy approach, because of its existentialist perspective, believes that individuals can actualize themselves, because of its phenomenological perspective, believes that individuals are special and unique, and because of its holistic perspective, believes that individuals constitute a whole both within themselves and with their environments. In the light of these beliefs, the Gestalt therapy approach considers the individual from a much more humane, flexible, and creative point of view than all other therapy approaches. At the same time, by utilizing years of accumulated knowledge from various former theories, perspectives, and therapy approaches and by integrating them into itself, Gestalt therapy offers a wide range of rich methods for the field of psychotherapy.

2

PSYCHOLOGICAL HEALTH

Like all other living beings, the two intrinsic characteristics of human beings are survival and growth (Perls 1973, 7). In order to survive and grow to maturity, people have to meet every kind of physical, psychological, and social need from the environment. As long as a need of any kind does not surface, the person or organism is in balance. The state of balance can be called homeostasis. However, as the organism has needs of every kind, this balance, or homeostasis, does not last for long. For instance, when the organism becomes aware of its thirst, hunger, or loneliness, in order to be able to restore the balance, it acts to resolve it. The organism falls back to homeostasis when the need is met and continues to be in this state until another need emerges. The organisms' being aware of its needs and taking action to satisfy them to restore homeostasis is called organismic self-regulation.

In the Gestalt approach, it is believed that all organisms are naturally self-regulating (Perls et al. 1951/1996, 294). By innately possessing the mechanism of self-regulation, a healthy organism is able to meet its needs and differentiate what is beneficial and what is harmful. In other words, a healthy person is able to notice which foods, people, situations, stimulants, etc., are nutritive and which are poisonous. In addition to that, each organism's self-regulation process is unique, and this process is influenced by both internal and environmental factors (Clarkson and Mackewn 1993, 48). For this reason, it is wrong to say "through self-regulation an organism can meet its needs always in the best possible way." For example, we will not be able to satisfy our needs if we are extremely thirsty in surroundings where there is no water or whilst starving refusing to eat in order to lose weight or furthermore avoiding to speak to anyone by saying, "I don't want to burden anyone with my worries" despite feeling lonely. In these situations, our self- regulation mechanism provides the strength to endure until the conditions are favorable and, at the same time, directs us to satisfy our needs in the best possible way within the given circumstances. On the other hand, if needs are not satisfied for a considerable time, the self-regulation mechanism of the organism is disrupted, which leads to physical and psychological illness and the development and the growth of the organism being interrupted.

Perls (1969, 28) indicated that neither plants nor animals but only people interrupt their own growth and development. Although Perls, in line with other therapeutic approaches, used the term *neurosis* for psychological problems, as psychological problems are the result of the organism's interrupting its own growth and development, he emphasized that "growth disorders" may be a more appropriate term to use for psychological problems.

In order to survive and grow, it is necessary for a person

   a.   to realize his/her needs
   b.   to determine the environmental circumstances
   c.   to put his/her needs and the environmental circumstances
        in harmony

Otherwise, when one of these three provisions is spoiled, the person cannot meet his/her needs and lose health. According to the Gestalt approach, both individual needs and environmental circumstances are highly important for psychological health. As psychological disturbances are results of the unsatisfied needs of a person, it is not appropriate to use the term *disease* for psychological disorders because the term *disease* implies that it is the person him/herself that is problematic. The Gestalt approach suggests that it is the disharmony between the person and his/her environment that causes ill health. Therefore, instead of disease, the use of expressions such as *disharmony* or *dis-ease* for psychological problems is preferred (Korb et al. 1989, 44).

Characteristics of a Healthy Person

The Gestalt approach emphasizes that psychologically healthy people are the ones who can take responsibility, actualize themselves, and who are authentic and mature. These characteristics of healthy people supplement one another rather than operating independently. Now we are going to expound on each one:

Healthy People Can Take Responsibility

According to the Gestalt approach, each person is responsible for his/her senses, emotions, thoughts, behaviors, needs, and knowing how to meet those needs. This perspective is based on the belief that each person is able to respond to psychological and physiological needs immediately and fully and has the freedom to give the reaction he/she wants to (Korb et al. 1989, 50). In other words, a person can determine his/her own values, make his/her own decisions, and display the appropriate action by identifying what is important and relevant for him/herself. To emphasize this point, Perls (1969/1992, 1973) interpreted the word *responsibility* as *response-ability* in his various writings.

However, some people carry the thought that they do not have the ability to respond. This derives from the belief that they are incapable of meeting their needs and acting on free will. This type of person tends to avoid responsibility by saying, "You know society will not permit this," "Although I do not agree with it, one has to obey the rules of society," "Society would not approve." These people expect society either to satisfy their needs or to give them the permission to satisfy their own needs. They blame relatives or others because of their needs. They avoid taking responsibility through self-pity, shouting, or emotional blackmail. Such expressions as "It is my partner who is not talking to me," "They asked very difficult questions in the exam," "That person started the fight first" serve as good examples to demonstrate how they push responsibility onto others or to the situation, and thus justify themselves. To a certain degree, they do have a point; however, by thinking in this pattern, they deny their own role in the occurrence of the problem and push themselves to a "helpless" position. In this way, they frequently play the "poor me game" (Korb et al. 1989, 63).

Generally, the situations where we have the most difficulty in taking responsibility for our feelings, thoughts, and behaviors is when our needs and desires are not in harmony with those of the people we consider important. In such situations, instead of taking the responsibility to clearly say they cannot meet these needs from the start, some people would either try to meet the demands and expectations of others reluctantly and feel bad or would blame and criticize the other persons for their demands and expectations and feel bad again. This is another form of the "poor me" game. The people who play the "poor me" game believe they are "victimized" by others, and they feel an "obligation" to meet other people's demands and expectations. However, one who is capable of taking responsibility and responding accordingly can give relevant explanations about why he/she cannot fulfill others' expectations and also will not blame others when his/her own needs are left unfulfilled.

Taking responsibility is quite an ordeal for humankind in general, and without a shadow of a doubt, one cannot be responsible for everything that happens within the environment. On the other hand, we are responsible for our actions, thoughts, emotions, and choices. People who take responsibility would not say, "See what happened to me," but would rather say, "See what happened to me, and I choose to do thus," or would not say, "He made me furious, and I could not control myself and beat him," but would rather say, "I got furious, and chose to beat him" (or, better, "I chose to control myself"). By acknowledging that "on this occasion I choose to behave in this way," the person gives him/herself the freedom to choose to behave in the same way or in a different way on another occasion. Otherwise, if we allow another person to determine our way of behaving and refuse to take responsibility, we limit our freedom and put ourselves in a helpless and weak position. Only by noticing what we do and taking personal responsibility for our actions we are able to develop the "ability to respond differently," gain freedom, and build self-confidence (Clarkson and Mackewn 1993, 61).

Healthy People Can Actualize Themselves

The concept of self-actualization was first articulated by Kurt Goldstein in the late 1930s. He coined this concept during the war years when he observed how people who had a brain damage showed eagerness to recover and improve their lives despite all that happened (Korb et al. 1989). Self-actualization doesn't mean to have the most supreme capabilities considered as "perfect" by others, but it means to be able to make full use of existing capabilities and potential. For example, a person who has actualized him/herself is not the most pretty, most successful, most diligent person, or the one who has the highest status. A person who has actualized him/herself accepts him/herself as he/she is. He/she is aware of his/her features, abilities, skills, and wishes. Maybe he/she is not the best but is aware of his/her beautiful sides. Maybe he/she is not the most successful, but he/she is very good at his/her areas of success and is able to enjoy his/her successes. Accepting oneself as one is and the quest to make the most out of what one is rather than what one wishes to be would prevent the organism from expecting perfection, which is both unrealistic and counter to organismic goals (Korb et al. 1989, 51). Hence, when one tries to actualize the "impossible" with a perfectionist attitude, one will not be actualizing oneself but a self- image (Perls 1973, 99). People who actualize not themselves but their self-images focus on surface-based values of physical appearance, grades, diplomas, status, and money, and even if they manage to achieve those, they are still unhappy because there is always a more perfect one out there. Being admired and appreciated by others with a sense of security is what these people find most important of all. Instead of trying to find out their own features, abilities, skills, and desires, they prefer to actualize the demands and ideals outlined by others. One of the areas where this is commonly practiced is related with the choice of profession. Some parents put pressure on their children by saying, "I always wanted to become a doctor, but I could not. Being a doctor is the best choice for you, and you will also look after us when we get older," or "Computer sciences are on the rise. Better become a computer engineer," or "You are a girl, you should go into teaching as it's the best profession for a girl. Besides you will have many days off." Overwhelmed by the pressure by their parents, adolescents tend to follow their parents' occupational choices and therefore cannot actualize themselves.

Healthy People Are Authentic

Authenticity means being open to one's own inner life and organizing the external world according to the inner experience (Korb et al. 1989, 52). An authentic person can choose freely how to express him/herself by being aware of his/her own self, others, and the conditions in general. That is, an authentic person would not act merely on his/her inner voice but also pay attention to the environment and act on his/her sole discretion. To give a good example, some people, for the sake of honesty, have the urge to say everything that comes into their mind without taking into account what others will feel about it. This is not authenticity. Authenticity is to determine what, when, and how to say or even whether to say it or not by bearing in mind both other people and environmental conditions. An authentic person can open up to others in a sincere, natural, and spontaneous way, and expresses him/herself as he/she is. Croker (1999, 242) states that the authentic person is the "author of his/her own life." Hence, the authentic person is unique and like only him/herself.

Healthy People Are Mature

Maturity is to have the ability to support oneself when necessary (Korb et al. 1989, 47). It is from the warmth of the mother's womb that a person gets the initial support in order to grow and develop. Later, his/her mother's milk and people who nursed him/her provide the support for his/her physical, mental, and social development. In time, with increasing capacity, skills, and knowledge, his/her dependency level decreases, and he/she acquires the skill to stand on his/her own two feet both socially and psychologically.

Maturation, or in other words, achieving self-support, is never an easy process and usually creates stress. The maturation process is about shifting away from the comfort zone of familiarity toward the territory of the unknown, which means taking risks, and this is always daunting. The process of maturation is an ongoing one because life is full of new events, new demands, and new relationships, and newness leads to anxiety and fear. Despite feeling anxious and fearful, mature people carry the strength to encourage themselves, keep calm, and move forward. As they are not incessantly "in need" of other people's approval and support as in childhood, they can rely on themselves and take the risk when they lack external support. On the other hand, immature people only focus on the experience of fear and anxiety whenever they encounter a novelty. They try to control the future and want assurance that something bad is not going to happen. As the future is unpredictable, they immobilize themselves. Due to the fear of losing other people's love, approval, and support, such people neither make their own decisions nor act alone. Perls (1969, 4) wrote the so- called Gestalt prayer to underline the significance of growing up to be a mature person being capable of self-support.

Gestalt Prayer

I do my thing and you do your thing.

I am not in this world to live up to your expectations, And you are not in this world to live up to mine.

You are you, and I am I,

And if by chance we find each other, it's beautiful. If not, it can't be helped.

Many people criticized Perls for placing too much emphasis on self-support and expressing it as a Gestalt prayer and regarded this attitude as exaggerated. Frankly, at first sight, this prayer may seem exaggerated. Yet this prayer should not be interpreted as meaning that Perls "only" emphasized the self-support feature of the person in the Gestalt approach. It must be borne in mind that the Gestalt approach addresses the person and the environment as a whole and psychological health is defined according to the harmony between the person and his/her environment. On the other hand, Clarkson and Mackewn (1993, 62) noted that according to the Gestalt therapy approach, self-support and maturity is not just about a person's self-confidence and isolation from others but, on the contrary, is also about being in relation with others as a "part of social life."

In brief, a psychologically healthy individual

- is aware of his/her own needs and willing to fulfill them,
- is self-accepting of all positive and negative aspects of him/

herself,is honest and sincere with him/herself and the environment,

- is able to ensure active contact with the environment,
- is considerate and sensitive toward his/her environment,
- is able to protect and support him/herself against the pressures of others,
- is able to take responsibility for his/her choices,
- is open to new experiences and ideas,
- has self-respect and self-confidence.

Without a doubt, it is not always easy for the person to achieve the aforementioned points. Yet a healthy individual does not quail at the possible adversities to be met when experiencing difficulties.

Factors Causing Mental Health Deterioration

According to the Gestalt approach, there are many factors causing mental health to deteriorate, or in other words, causing disharmony. Both Perls and other Gestalt therapists define the factors that act out in the disharmony between the organism and the environment in different ways and emphasize different points. Yet in Gestalt theory, the main factors that play a role in the deterioration of psychological health can be summarized as follows:

- Incomplete experience cycle
- Dysfunctional contact styles
- Unfinished business
- Unresolved impasses
- Unintegrated poles

These factors are discussed in detail in different chapters of this book. Certainly the intensity and the influence of these factors in the deterioration of psychological health vary from person to person. The intensity and the influence of these factors determine the level of the psychological problem, or in other words, the level of neurosis.

Layers of Psychological Problems

In his model, in order to identify psychological problems, Perls (1969, 75–77) indicated five layers of neurosis. The first is the cliché layer. This level is about daily activities, which mainly involve brief chats and greetings, and has no correspondence to the actual emotions of the person. Real contact is not experienced in this layer as the person behaves according to introjected cultural values. The second is the role layer. Perls suggested that this layer could also be named the "Eric Berne" or "Sigmund Freud" layer as both therapy approaches deal with neurosis on this level. At the role level, the person uses the contact styles he/she learned over and over again and behaves according to one of the selected roles as "an important person," "a helpless victim," "a kind little girl," "a devoted mother," etc. The third is the impasse layer. In this layer, there is a conflict between the healthy side that wants to complete the unfinished business and the side that wants to avoid distress. Most people would avoid this conflict as experiencing the impasse is an uncomfortable situation that leads to feelings of anxiety, confusion, and being stuck. To escape from experiencing the impasse, the person usually tries to change the persons around him/her. The fourth layer is called the implosive layer, also referred as the death layer. This layer brings a state of paralysis of opposing forces. The person believes that if he/she expresses him/herself to others, he/she will lose the control and love of others. Trying to keep everything inside him/her and under control also leads to bodily tensions. The fifth is the explosive layer. In this layer, if the individual faces the anxiety, confusion, and feeling of being stuck experienced in the third level and the paralysis experienced in the fourth level, he/she will come back to life. The person begins to feel and experience emotions and be active. The confrontation on this level may lead to four types of explosion. If the impasse is linked with death or loss, the explosion will be experienced as grief; if the impasse is linked with sexuality, the explosion will be experienced as orgasm; if linked with incapacity to express positive feelings, it will be experienced as joy, and if linked with the incapacity to express negative feelings, it will be experienced as anger. The intensity of the explosion depends on the level of internal accumulation. In therapy the aim is to reach the fifth layer as it is believed that one can start to grow and develop only after the explosion.

The Goals of the Therapy

In every therapy approach, the goal of the therapy can be classified in three groups, and these are the ultimate goal, common goal, and personal goal. Definitely, the ultimate goal of all therapy approaches is to help the person to be and remain psychologically healthy. According to the Gestalt approach, the ultimate goal is to create people who are able to meet their needs and have harmonious relations with the environment without hindering their growth and development.

Through the awareness-raising process, helping the individual to take his/her own responsibility and to change his/her life is the common purpose of all Gestalt practices (Evans 1999). In reaching these goals, first, clients realize "how they are" in terms of their own emotions, thoughts, behaviors, bodies, and needs; second, they take the responsibility for choosing to "be like this," and third, they understand that they can change their life "by behaving differently," if they want.

The individual goal of the therapy is determined according to the complaints and needs of the client as well as the opinions of the therapist. The personal goal of Gestalt practice ranges from self- actualization to overcoming symptoms of insomnia, attention deficit, fear and psychogenic pains, etc. Therefore, the Gestalt therapy approach is applicable not only to the individuals who experience severe psychological problems but to everyone who wants to understand and actualize themselves as well.

Clinical Applications

In general, the Gestalt therapy approach is used for all types of neurotic, psychotic, and personality disorders listed under psychiatric classifications and achieves successful results on its own or together with other therapy approaches and medical treatments. Some of the problem areas in which the Gestalt therapy approach is found effective are given below:

- Phobias (Johnson and Smith 1997; Evans 1999)
- Performance anxiety (Garcia, Baker, DeMoya 1999; Wingfield 1999)

- Anxiety disorders (Daş 2004)
- Depression and perfectionism (Shepherd 1970, 234–235)
- Crisis situations and adaptation problems (Simkin and Yontef 1984)
- Post-traumatic stress disorder (Cohen 2003)
- Psychosomatic problems (migraine, ulcers, neck and back pain, etc.) (Yontef 1993,165)
- Hypertension (Serok 2000, 79–88)
- Personality disorders (Shub 1994b; Shub 1999; Yontef 1993, 419–489)
- Alcoholism (Carlok, Glaus, and Shaw 1992; Clemens 1997) and gambling addiction (Shub 1998b)
- Sexual problems (Yolaç and Tuğrul 1991; Tuğrul 1998, 1999)
- Marital problems (Zinker 1994; Wheeler and Backman 1994; Kempler 1978; Brown 1998)
- Schizophrenia (Serok 2000, 117–156; Harris 1992)
- Childhood problems (Oaklender 1992; Root 1996)
- Adolescence problems (McConville 1995; Serok 2000, 156–163)
- Geriatric problems (Woldt and Stein 1997; Serok 2000, 103–114)

The Gestalt therapy approach has been effectively practiced to overcome organizational problems of companies and institutions (Nevis, Lancourt, and Vassallo 1996; Nevis 1998) and to enhance the performance of executives and employees working in various sectors (Daş 2003a), students (Polster and Polster 1974), health care workers and artists (Huckabay 1992), as well as for personal development purposes.

As can be seen, the Gestalt therapy approach can be applied for various purposes. In order to attain a set of goals, individual, couple, family, or group based therapies are offered. The needs of the client determine the type of therapy to be applied. Each type of therapy has its own advantages and disadvantages. For instance, individual therapy practice is favorable for privacy: the client has all the attention to him/ herself, the session intervals are planned in line with client's needs, and the client expresses his/her problems only to the therapist rather than to everyone involved, as in a group therapy session. On the other hand, couples and family therapy practices are favorable for enabling work with more than one person who has relationship problems with each other, to observe contact styles in the relationship during the therapy session, to help the couple to experience new contact styles together, and through trial.

By taking into account the person and the environment as a whole and making the relationship between the person and the environment its focal point, Gestalt therapy, in comparison to other therapeutic approaches, is the most appropriate approach in group therapies (Frew 1997). The Gestalt approach outlines different types of group therapies for various purposes. These groups can be presented under four main headings: (A) individual oriented groups, (B) group processed oriented groups, (C) personal development oriented groups, and (D) training oriented groups. Below are the details of the group practices.

Group Practices

a. Individual Oriented Groups

By applying it to a group of people ranging from ten to a couple of hundred, Perls commenced with individual oriented groups at a time when the Gestalt therapeutic approach was initially being conceptualized (Latner 1986, 143). In particular, the hot seat technique is used in such groups (Polster Polster 1974, 286). It is based on one-to-one work between a volunteer group member and the therapist in a group setting. In classical Gestalt practices, the group member, in the middle, would focus on his/her dreams, fantasies, expectations, facial expressions, and gestures or other characteristics while the rest of the group would follow passively (Wheeler 1998, 102). Some therapists also involve other group members in the process and let the group member in the center contact with and receive feedback from them, if necessary (Clarkson and Mackewn 1993, 131). In some group practices, the topic is determined by the group and the therapist in advance, and the therapist specifically works on this topic with the volunteer member. As well as lasting for a couple of hours or days, individual oriented group work mostly runs for several weeks on given specific times as a closed group.

The chief goal of the individual oriented groups is psychological change. As the intervention of the therapist is on a personal level, the interpersonal relation is limited to the relationship between the client and the therapist (Kitzler 1994). In these practices, the group is used to enhance the impact of individual work. Some therapists suggest that such groups are not different than individual therapy and thus can be called "individual work in front of the group." However, one-to- one work in a group is different than a private session and has certain advantages (Polster and Polster 1974, 286–287). The first advantage is that by having an "audience," the client feels him/herself within a supportive group or "community," and this provides a meaningful deep experience. The second advantage is to give an opportunity to the other members to raise their own awareness by observing the client and the therapist. Third, the person in the center can get help from other group members when necessary. Finally, the fourth advantage is that far more people are reached via group therapy than are via individual therapy.

These groups, as well as their advantages, also have some disadvantages. Although these practices take place in front of the group, the communication and interaction among group members is neglected because the actual work is on a one-to-one basis, between the client and the therapist. Consequently, the client in the middle is unable to be aware of the characteristics of his/her contact with others, nor are the other members able to benefit from the group as they are not allowed to express themselves (Latner 1986, 143). Another disadvantage is that the therapist is unable to receive any support from group members because of doing all the work alone and taking all of the responsibility. This leads to a disruption of the dialogue relation, which is fundamental to the Gestalt approach. Because of these disadvantages, later Gestalt therapists moved away from this model of Perls's toward "experiential" or "process" type group practices (Wheeler 1998, 103). Today, individual oriented work is seldom practiced.

b. Group Process Oriented Groups

On one hand, members of the process oriented groups focus on the spoken topic by referring to their own life experiences and, on the other hand, observe and share the experiences of other group members and become engaged in the process. The "floating hot seat" technique is used in these groups. Even though the therapist is working face to face with one person at a time in the floating hot seat technique as the other members have the right to participate in the process, the person in the hot seat and its location may change frequently, so the hot seat actually "floats" around the group (Polster and Polster 1974, 287). Group process oriented practices are based on the belief that the group is a whole and the structure of the group is more and different than just its constituent members. In other words, the group is not merely a crowd of people, but a psychosocial milieu that influences and in return is influenced by the emotions, attitudes, and behaviors of the members in the system (Kepner 1994, 7).

In group process oriented groups (a) focus is on the group experience, (b) the aim is to raise group awareness, (c) there is active contact among the members, and (d) various Gestalt methods and techniques are guided by the therapist (Zinker 1977, 161). In these groups, members are supported by the therapist to express their personal inner experience and share it with the other members of the group. While the therapist, as a catalyst, ensures various individual themes are integrated within group experience, members become aware of how they influence other members and are influenced by them in return.

In group oriented practices, the therapist works with the individual as well as with the group (Kitzler 1994). For this reason, it is possible to make interventions on three levels, the personal, interpersonal, and group level, during the practice. The interventions are made on thoughts, feelings, senses, etc., at the personal level; on projections, conflicts, confluences, etc., at the interpersonal level; and on group norms, culture, atmosphere, etc., at the group level. The level of interventions is determined according to the goals of the group. This type of Gestalt group practice achieves a higher advantage over other therapy approaches by intervening on all three levels, whereas other approaches either intervene only on one or two levels (Frew 1997). Focusing on the individual awareness that is achieved during the session makes it easy for the members to make contact with each other, and this is another advantage of group-oriented practices. This type of group practice enables each member to develop self-expression skills as well as a better self-understanding. Moreover, group sharing enables the members to have a better understanding of one another and their interactions (Passons 1975, 68).

c. Personal Development Oriented Groups

Anyone willing to know about him/herself and to have better relations both with him/herself and with other persons around him/her may participate in personal development oriented groups. Such groups are also known as "therapy for normal people" (Kepner 1994). This type of group can be practiced anywhere, with anyone, and at any time, whether planned or spontaneous. For instance, Polster and Polster (1974, 292–301) mentioned how they performed a group practice at a patisserie with people who were gathered there by coincidence. In such practices, there is an interactive relation between the therapist and the group members (Feder and Ronal 1994). In some of the personal development oriented group practices, the topic to work on is determined according to the needs of the group, while in others, it is determined according to the needs of the individual. Also there are some other group practices that are organized as workshops, where various techniques are used according to certain preidentified themes (Feder and Ronall 1994). Because of having a common purpose as a group, this kind of personal development practice provides a sense of equality among the members, a quicker achievement of group unity, and a deeper experience (Zinker 1977, 168).

In some personal development oriented group practices, the focus is on artistic activities, bodily expression and movements. Both in artistic activities (such as painting, sculpture, mask making, and fabric or wood coloring) and bodily expressions through movements and dancing, it is not the artistic or dancing talents but expressing oneself and the raising of awareness that is important. In all artistic- and movement-based practices, the meanings of the "creations" are specific to the person who created them. Compared to the practices where only verbal expressions are used, the aforementioned practices provide an easier, faster, and deeper awareness (Rapp 1994, 87).

The point of view that lies at the basis of artistic practices is that physical, mental, and emotional characteristics, needs, unfinished business, impasses, poles, and resistances of the person will be reflected symbolically in the artistic creation (Ryhne 1984, 5). Movement and dance practices, where feelings, thoughts, needs, and desires are expressed via the body, are very helpful in the integration of the body, the mind and the soul, which is one of the fundamentals of the Gestalt approach (Tyler 1994, 104). In some practices preidentified musical pieces are used, whereas in some others, a variety of rhythms and musical instruments or oral melodies are preferred. During these practices, the use of music enables the comfortable emergence of body movements and also helps the members to integrate within and with the environment easily. Also, in some practices members are encouraged to accompany bodily movements with vocal sounds. The use of the body and the voice together plays a significant role especially in becoming aware of the senses and the feelings (Rebelliot 2004).

Personal development oriented Gestalt groups can be organized in various ways. For example, some groups may last for a few days, whereas some others may be organized to meet on a particular day and time for longer periods. Marathon groups are another way of practicing. These are residential groups, where the sessions last for extra-long hours. Mintz (1994) described the marathon groups as more favorable than other practices, as they give opportunity (a) to be aware of similarities among other members of the group in a secure, caring, and warm environment, (b) to move away from daily life and focus more on here and now, and (c) to release the blocked energy easily by working on the emotional problems several times and in different ways.

d. Training Oriented Groups

These groups are developed in order to present an applied and experiential model to the trainees when teaching the Gestalt therapy approach (Ronall 1994). The purpose of training oriented groups is to teach the students the Gestalt therapy approach both on perceptual and cognitive levels and also to help them develop by raising individual awareness. The students' experiencing Gestalt concepts via awareness also contributes to their personal growth. The leader of such groups will act like both as a trainer and as a therapist (Feder 1994).

These groups may have different structures, but in all training groups, four fields are covered (Ronall 1994). These are as follows:

a. *Big group (group-as-a-whole) work.* This work involves providing support for all members to express themselves individually by focusing on the present. Additionally, various exercises on the theme of the group are worked out.

b. *Theoretical work.* The leader gives lectures on Gestalt theory and concepts, and related practices are performed.

c. *Small group work.* Each member takes the role of a therapist, a client, and an observer alternately. They come together to develop their therapeutic skills by practicing therapy and receiving supervision.

d. *Evaluation of the process.* The aim of such work is to integrate the group experiences with didactic knowledge, as well as activating information process and increasing group unity.

In such practices, basic Gestalt concepts such as "awareness," "dreams," "contact styles," or specific issues such as "adolescence problems," "personality disorders," etc., or "Gestalt therapy" in general can be chosen as a theme to work on. The training oriented groups may vary in duration. Some training oriented groups may meet on a particular day of the week for a couple of hours, while others hold meetings for three to five days at certain intervals or two-to-four-week- long residential groups might be arranged.

Consequently, the point of view of the Gestalt therapy approach to psychological health has brought many innovations to the field of psychotherapy. Firstly, by not using the term *illness*, Gestalt therapy rejects the labeling of people and instead emphasizes the growth and development capacity of people by using expressions such as *disorders*, *dis-ease*, or *disharmony*. Secondly, unlike other approaches, the Gestalt therapy approach asserts that the problem is not in the person or the environment but in the person/environment field and therefore has a broader perspective toward psychological health. Thirdly, the Gestalt approach does not see the client as a "victim" who needs to be "cured" by a therapist but rather sees the client as an active participant who has the necessary potential to meet his/her own needs, who can take responsibility and who is capable of self-actualization. Fourthly, by being applicable to every kind of psychological problem as well as to everyone who is in search of self-knowledge and self-improvement, the Gestalt approach brought another innovation to the field of psychotherapy. Finally, incorporating art, dance, and music into the therapy with the aim of facilitating body-mind-soul integrity is another innovation.

3

THERAPEUTIC RELATIONSHIP AND THE GESTALT THERAPIST

According to the Gestalt approach, the essence of therapy is the contact between two people (Clarkson and Mackewn 1993, 87). In other words, therapy is the relation between two "real" people. Gestalt perspective believes that growth and change can be possible only within the context of a relationship. The client can only start to question his/her personal life, entitle it, and to be aware of it if he/she believes that the therapist is also "real," just like him/her. Again according to the Gestalt approach, the healing process depends neither on the therapist nor on the client but on what is going on between the therapist and the client that is on the dialogue between them (Mackewn 1997, 80). Joyce and Sills (2003, 41) have indicated that the most important characteristics in terms of change and growth were the creation of a safe environment in addition to the therapeutic relation established during the dialogue.

In its most general sense, dialogue is a conversation between two people. However, in the Gestalt approach, dialogue that is regarded as the basis of growth and change is not just any ordinary conversation but a dialogue that depends on the existential encounter between the therapist and the client. The concept of "existential dialogue" was proposed by Martin Buber (1958) and depends on I-Thou relation. Existential dialogue is the meeting of two people, each with different styles of existence and different needs who accept their differences and respect each other (Yontef 1993, 203). In this human-to-human encounter, while both sides are sharing their own inner experiences, they are mutually affected and react to each other.

As the Gestalt approach considers the dialogic relationship between the therapist and the client the most important healing factor of the therapy, this is one of its most distinguishing differences of Gestalt therapy from other therapy approaches. Perls (1947/1992, 231) criticized the psychoanalytic approach on this subject as follows: Transference work and the interpretations related to it, which is the focus of the psychoanalytic approach, decreases the client's responsibility, encourages transference, makes human-to-human contact difficult, and strengthens cognitive defenses. Perls has also opposed some other approaches that focus only on behaviors and those that claim that application of certain techniques is necessary for therapeutic success. The dialogic relation emphasized in the Gestalt approach is a horizontal relation, not a vertical one (Yontef 1993, 212). In vertical relations, the parties are not at an equal level and the therapist has an authoritarian attitude and tries to determine what is good or bad for the client, what he/she should do and how it should be done. The therapy approaches where vertical relations prevail use the medical model. In the medical model, there is a "patient," an "illness," and an "expert" who heals. In a horizontal relationship, on the other hand, the therapist has no need to display an authoritative attitude, to play a neutral doctor role, or to act like an expert hiding behind his/her mask. The therapist expresses him/herself and shares his/her responses and reactions with the client in an authentic way (Clarkson and Mackewn 1993, 88).

Jacops (1989), Hycner (1991), and Yontef (1993, 202–237) consider the Gestalt therapy approach as a dialogic relation, that is, as I-Thou relationship. During therapy, creating the appropriate atmosphere for the establishment of I-Thou relationship, or in other words, to enable a human-to-human contact and interaction is one of the most important responsibilities of the therapist (Perls 1973, 112). The characteristics of I-Thou relationship can be explained as follows.

Characteristics of the Dialogic Relationship

The characteristics of the dialogic relationship can be grouped under four headings such as the therapist's acceptance of the client's way of being, the therapist's presentation of him/herself actively, the therapist's participation in the therapeutic process, and the therapist's being open and willing for a sincere communication. Actually, the four characteristics are not separate from each other, but rather they are complementary to each other and intertwined with each other. The purpose of dealing with them separately above is to emphasize the different facets of the dialogic relationship.

Accepting the Client's Way of Being

According to the Gestalt approach, the most important thing that a therapist can offer to his/her client is a willingness to listen and talk to him/her without any expectations, judgments, or evaluations. Here, acceptance of the client's way of being means that the therapist listens to what the client has done and what he/she has experienced and shows an effort to understand them. For many people, the therapist is the first and only person who takes their thoughts, feelings, needs, and experiences seriously and who listens and tries to understand them. In such a relationship, the client could feel that no matter what he/she does, be, or think, he/she is still someone who is valuable and lovable. For the client to like and appreciate him/herself and to gain awareness of him/herself can only be possible if the client believes that the therapist is accepting him/her as he/she is (Zinker 1977, 60). On the other hand, therapist's acceptance of the client's way of being does not mean that he/she is approving and supporting everything the client does (Joyce and Sills 2003, 46). Furthermore, some of client's behavior (such as using substances or showing violence against family members) could be behaviors that the therapist never approves. Sometimes the therapist may have negative feelings for the unapproved actions of the client but always remembers that the client is behaving this way because he or she "cannot manage to do better." While the therapist is trying to listen to and understand the client, he/she tries to hear not only what the client is saying but what he/she is not saying and what he/she is not aware of (Yontef 1993,

222). For example, in a case where the client repeatedly talks about how lazy he/she is, the therapist might recognize how industrious he/she is in some circumstances. In such cases, the therapist shares with the client the characteristics that he/she recognized while listening. During the dialogic relationship, therapist encourages the client to express him/herself fully. The therapist's respecting the thoughts, feelings, and behaviors of the client leads the client to start respecting him/herself.

Presenting Him/Herself Actively

According to the Gestalt approach, the most important tool within a therapeutic relationship is the therapist's presenting him/herself actively (Yontef 1993, 210). During the session, the therapist is ready for the client every moment with his/her full attention and vitality. In other words, the therapist enters the session with his/her whole being and gives him/herself fully to the therapeutic experience. While the therapist tries to understand the client using his/her skills, training, observations, and intuitions, the therapist also tries to be aware of his/her own feelings, thoughts, and behaviors related to the relationship with the client and what the client has been telling. The Gestalt therapist who is in a dialogic relationship does not take on a neutral and objective role but, on the contrary, exposes him/herself fully with all his/her being and as he/she is. In other words, the Gestalt therapist does not "play a role," does not "try to leave a particular impression," and does not behave "as if." A therapist who tries to be seen neutral when very concerned or who tries to look calm when excited seems present but is not present actively (Yontef 1993, 222).

A therapist, who is exposing him/herself with all his being and as he/she is, establishes an authentic relationship with the client. The opposite of establishing an authentic relationship is establishing a strategic one (Joyce and Sills 2003, 45). According to Buber (1958/1984, 16–18), an authentic relationship depends on I-Thou relationship while the strategic relationship depends on I-It one. In an I-It relationship, we regard other people as objects and try to affect, control, and manipulate them. Likewise we feel that they are also affecting us and trying to control and manipulate us. A therapist who is in I-It, or in other words, in a strategic relationship, relates to the client not in the "here" and "now" as should be the case with the Gestalt approach but with all his/her knowledge, prejudices, rights, wrongs, and expectations from his/her past. Many people are in such a relationship with others during their daily life in order to satisfy their needs, wishes and plans. Whereas the therapist who establishes an authentic relationship with the client, sees him/her in the "here" and "now" as he/she is, listens sincerely, does not try to place the client somewhere that is familiar from his/her previous experiences, and presents him/herself honestly. This open and accepting style of the therapist invites the clients also to be open and accepting. The natural and spontaneous reactions of the therapist accelerate the development of a trust relationship between the therapist and the client (Korb et al. 1989, 110).

Participating in the Therapeutic Process

In order to participate in the therapy process, it is necessary for the therapist to regard therapy not only from his/her point of view but also from the client's point of view as well as from the perspective of the relationship with the client (Joyce and Sills 2003, 47). The first condition of the therapist's participation in the therapeutic process is to accept the client as he/she is and to enter the client's phenomenological world with respect (Yontef 1993, 221). In order to avoid a disrespectful entry to the client's world, the therapist "brackets" his/her points of views and beliefs. This means that the therapist does not judge the client in terms of his/her own view points and beliefs, does not try to impose them on the client, and does not try to convince him/her. Instead the therapist tries to look at the client's world empathically from where the client stands, with his/her eyes and as he/she is. Since feelings are universal and since everybody has feelings of loneliness, sadness, anger, joy, excitement, anxiety, etc., it is not difficult for the therapist to empathize with client's feelings and to enter his/her world. However, if the therapist is not at peace with his/her own feelings, for example, if the therapist is afraid of his/her own anger or scared of showing sadness by crying, then he/she cannot be empathic with the client's expressions of emotions and may even obstruct him/her. This makes it imperative that the Gestalt therapists themselves should go through therapy themselves. On the other hand, the Gestalt therapist should take into consideration the fact that everybody can experience different feelings under different circumstances and show different reactions in different situations. Hence, while the therapist is trying to understand the client's experiences, the therapist should share what he/she understood and check with the client whether or not he/she understood correctly.

The second condition of the therapist's participation in the therapy is to be aware of his own phenomenology, that is, to be aware of his/her own experiences, feelings, and reactions regarding the client's feelings, behaviors, or what he/she tells during therapy. In other words, while the therapist is trying to listen, observe, and understand the client, he/she also tries to listen, observe, and understand him/herself. In the dialogic relationship, once the therapist becomes aware of his/her own experiences, feelings, and reactions, then he/she shares them with the client. This can be done at cognitive, emotional, bodily levels or as a nonverbal communication (Joyce and Sills 2003, 48). During the sharing, for example, regarding the thoughts and beliefs of the client, the therapist can make statements such as "I see that you believe you should not ask for help on this subject," "I understand that you think your mother behaves this way because she does not love you." When deemed necessary, the therapist can express his/her feelings arising from what the client is telling as "To see how sad you feel about your friend's comments made me feel sad also" or "I was very much effected with your facial expression when you were talking about your success in the latest exam." Emotional sharing can sometimes be achieved nonverbally with the tone of voice, way of sitting, way of looking, or with gestures and mimics.

In some cases, the therapist, in addition to his/her feelings, may wish to share his/her bodily reactions also and give messages such as "I realize that while listening to what happened between you and your husband, I hold my breath and worry," "What you are telling about your sister's illness filled my eyes with tears," or "If I were you, I would have become angry in such a situation." In other cases, the therapist may find it useful to give examples from his/her life that are similar to the situations or feelings that the client has experienced. Stern (1985) names the therapists' accompanying the client or conveying how he/she was affected with the client's experiences as "emotional accord." In a dialogical relationship, after sharing his/her own experiences, feelings, and reactions with the client, the therapist should also explore the feelings of the client about that sharing. Such sharing has a strong healing effect as they allow the client to experience his/her feelings easily during the therapy and as they make the client feel understood and accepted by the therapist. Furthermore, such sharing can also enable the deepening of the relationship between the therapist and the client. In this way, a new relationship, a new dance, is created during therapy where both sides are participating and affecting each other (Joyce and Sills 2003, 48). As the relationship between the therapist and the client is very important for the therapeutic process, one of the responsibilities of the therapist is to share his/her observations, feelings, and thoughts about this relationship with the client. In order to manage this, the therapist has to have the skill of going back and forth between his/her own world and that of the client and the ability to look at the relationship between them from a distance. A therapist with these skills can convey his/her observations, feelings, and thoughts to the client with remarks such as "I am aware that we have so far kept talking about others. What do you think can be preventing us from taking up a subject related to you?" or "I see that you are frequently asking, 'I don't know if you understand me?' "What is going on between us that makes you think that I might not understand you?" or "You are saying that you don't know what to do and you are not getting any benefit from the therapy. What do you expect me to do so you can benefit from therapy?" Such an approach allows the responsibility to be shared between the therapist and client about what is experienced in therapy and also makes it possible to investigate them without being judgmental. A joint acceptance of the responsibility of the relationship between the therapist and the client is different from many other therapy approaches in general and from the psychoanalytical approach where the responsibility of transference is on the client alone in particular.

Being Open and Willing to a Sincere Communication

In terms of a dialogic relationship, the therapist's being open and willing to sincerely share his/her observations, feelings, thoughts, or life experiences with the client is very crucial as the therapist takes a lot of risks by presenting him/herself as he/she is. In order to be open and willing to a sincere communication, the therapist has to have the courage to expose him/herself, trust what he/she experiences during the therapy, and respect what the client is experiencing (Yontef 1993, 223). On the other hand, therapist's having a sincere and open communication with the client does not mean that the therapist is going to tell his/her every feeling, every thought, every observation, or every memory that comes out during therapy to the client. There is no doubt that the therapist's sharing whatever comes to his/her mind with the client is not therapeutic, and it is very objectionable. To have the therapist convey his/her every reaction to the client can adversely affect the process of the client and even can stop it. It might lead the client to put him/herself aside, to focus on the therapist, to getting bored with what the therapist is saying, to get angry unnecessarily, and not to be able to express his/her feelings and experience them.

The therapist should only share those feelings, thoughts, observations, and experiences that he/she thinks could benefit and help the client (Yontef 1993, 223). In other words, the therapist should not communicate these to the client unless he/she has a valid reason. Another important point regarding sharing is when and how the therapist shares what he/she wants to share. For example, such sharing should not be made at the initial stages of the therapy. Furthermore, such sharing should be judged carefully with clients who are experiencing serious depression or anxiety, those who recently had a trauma, who are in a vulnerable state, and who are diagnosed with personality disorders. How to carry out the sharing should also be planned with attention to the needs of the client and what he/she is ready to hear.

However, there are no definite criteria about what, when, and how something should be shared, and all of these are determined according to the therapist's skill and experience. In conclusion, I-Thou dialogue to be established with the client is significant in terms of the following:

- It is essential in the establishment of an honest and reliable relationship during therapy.
- It is important for enabling the client to feel understood and accepted.

- Opening up of the therapist him/herself prevents the power struggle between the therapist and client.

- To have the therapist to expose him/herself sincerely and openly leads the client to take the therapist as a role model and to express him/herself sincerely and openly.

- It helps the client to accept feelings such as jealousy, sadness, anxiety, anger, etc., that he/she is either unaware of or refusing to acknowledge.

- It helps in revealing situations where the client fails to show a healthy reaction because of various reasons (such as getting angry when mistreated).

- Through the relationship established with the therapist, it enables the client to become aware of how he/she is establishing relationships with others.

When the client comes for therapy, he/she is in a distressed and troubled state and maybe expecting the therapist to solve his/her problems and take his/her responsibility and hence might have difficulty to adapt to an I-Thou relationship. In such a case, the therapist does not give up I-Thou dialogue. Instead, within I-Thou dialogue, the therapist helps the client to be aware of his/her expectations about the "inability to solve his/her problems" and "inability to take his/her own responsibility" and investigates the roots of such expectations (Sills et al. 1998, 20). In this way, the therapist, through I-Thou dialogue, enables the client to change without trying to change him/her (Yontef 1993, 217). In other words, I-Thou dialogue inevitably leads to change.

Characteristics of the Gestalt Therapist

In order to achieve successful results in therapy, besides the therapeutic relationship established with the client, the characteristics of the therapist also play a very important role. The characteristics of a Gestalt therapist can be summarized as observer, director, educator, catalyzer, and creative. Each of these characteristics of the Gestalt therapist is explained below.

The Gestalt Therapist Should Be an Observer

Gestalt therapy is an approach that focuses on the "here" and "now," that is, on what happens during the session and in the therapy room. Therefore, during therapy, may be even more attention is paid to what the client "does" as well as what he/she tells. Perls (1973, 177–179) has claimed that Gestalt therapy is an approach which "focuses on the obvious" and stated that "real communication is experienced beyond words." Hence, it is not sufficient to focus on what is being heard during therapy, as is the case in many other approaches, but in contrast, the therapist should pay attention to the bodily and non-verbal behavior of the client and observe them. In the Gestalt approach it is believed that particularly unrecognized feelings are expressed through different parts of the body, body movements and bodily functions (Mackewn 1999, 162). Hence, the therapist should have the skill to carefully observe the client's way of sitting and breathing, facial expressions, gestures and mimics, bodily and vocal changes.

The Gestalt Therapist Should Be a Director

One of the tasks of the therapist, using his/her clinical knowledge and experience, is to diagnose the client according to the Gestalt perspective, to decide what the client needs to achieve the goals set for the therapy, to evaluate the path taken during therapy, and to make plans about the issues to be covered and the techniques to be applied that could be useful in therapy. For this, the therapist should not always remain in I-Thou dialogue but, from time to time, following a strategic pattern, should also establish I-It dialogue. Jacobs (1989) has indicated that the dialogue during therapy should be carried out interchanging between I-Thou and I-It relationships. Particularly during the evaluations in the beginning of the therapy and at times of impasse, the therapist's being directive is important (Korb et al. 1989, 128). The therapist also has to direct the client to various exercises to raise awareness, to complete unfinished business, to integrate the polarities, to recognize bodily and nonverbal clues or to understand the messages given through dreams. On the other hand, the therapist should also have the necessary knowledge to decide on the possible diagnosis of the client according to the psychiatric classifications and whether or not the client needs medical help and when necessary should be able to direct the client to another expert. However, to the extent that it is possible, the therapist should conduct the therapy within I-Thou relationship and, when entered into an I-It relationship, should avoid taking an authoritarian attitude.

The Gestalt Therapist Should Be an Educator

One of the characteristics of Gestalt therapist is being an educator. The therapist may need to inform and give explanations to the client about the Gestalt perspective on topics such as the importance of needs, the need satisfaction cycle, styles of contact, unfinished business, personal responsibility, creative adjustment, etc. However, this should be done according to the client's needs, appropriate to his/her phenomenology, and within I-Thou dialogue, and such information should never be imposed to the client. The client should always have the right to accept or reject these information and explanations. According to the Gestalt approach, the most permanent way of learning is learning through experience. Hence, one of the therapist's tasks is to help the client to learn through experience. The Gestalt approach has a great variety of exercises developed for this purpose. Through these exercises, the client learns what his/her needs, modes of contact, resistances, etc., are. According to Perls (1973, 125), learning is "to see that something is possible." The therapist, therefore, in a dialogic relationship, by talking about his/her own feelings, thoughts or experiences becomes a model for the client and gives an opportunity to the client to see that he/she could also do them (Korb et al. 1989, 115). Similarly, as the client sees that the therapist is accepting him/her as he/she is; respects and takes seriously his/her feelings, thoughts, behaviors and needs, then he/she also starts to accept, respect and give importance to him/herself.

The Gestalt Therapist Should Be a Catalyzer

As mentioned before, one of underlying viewpoints of the Gestalt therapy approach is the phenomenological perspective. According to the phenomenological approach, what is important is not the generally accepted meaning of an incident, situation, experience, but their specific and unique meaning for that person at that moment and at that place

(Sills et al. 1998, 89). Another important viewpoint of Gestalt therapy approach is that "every person is responsible for their own lives" (Clarkson 1991, 24). Based on these two basic points of view of the Gestalt approach, one of the tasks of the therapist is while trying to understand the meaning of the feelings, thought, and experiences that are unique to the client, at the same time to increase the client's awareness level about his/her possible choices. In this sense, the therapist is not "helping" the client as in the general sense but acts as a catalyzer to enable the client to reach his/her goals (Korb et al. 1989, 122). In other words, the therapist does not suggest what the client should do, what to change and how to act, that is, the therapist does not impose his/her solutions or value judgments upon the client. Instead, the therapist, as a catalyzer, by enabling the client to be aware of and experience all his/her difficulties, impasses, polarities, and resistances, helps the client to find his/her own solutions and to take on his/her own responsibilities. According to the Gestalt approach, the only person to decide about what to do, what to change, and how to behave is the client him/herself, and he/she should be the one to take the responsibility for his/her decisions. The therapist does not decide for the client and, in this sense, doesn't take the client's responsibility (Yontef 1993, 266).

The Gestalt Therapist Should Be a Creator

In the Gestalt approach, there are an infinite number of experiments and strategies that can be applied during therapy. The therapist has to select the interventions that could be useful at that time, for that person, under that situation, and for that problem from his/her existing repertoire, to adapt them for the client, and if necessary, to create new ones (Zinker 1977, 55). There are no rules in the Gestalt approach that instruct the therapist to apply which interventions, when, to which client, in which situations, and for which problems. In other words there are no pre-prepared "prescriptions" or "package" programs in the Gestalt approach. Because of this, the therapist has to have a very vast exercise repertoire and also has to be very creative. Furthermore, in addition to creating experiments for the client, the therapist has to create the conditions and atmosphere within which the interventions can be carried out (Amendt-Lyon 2001). The creativity of the therapist also helps in bringing out the creative traits of the client.

In conclusion, the success of the Gestalt approach depends on the quality of the therapeutic relationship established between the therapist and the client and to the extent that the therapist has the characteristics mentioned above. When the Gestalt approach was first proposed, many people claimed that the success of the approach was due to the personality characteristics of Perls himself. Actually everybody who watched the film shots during his therapy sessions could easily see that he possessed all the mentioned characteristics of the therapist and more. Gestalt therapists go through a long and comprehensive therapy training in order to internalize the aforementioned characteristics. It is necessary to be an expert in one of the fields like psychology, psychological counseling, social work, or psychiatry in order to be accepted for the Gestalt therapy training. Gestalt therapists, besides the theoretical and technical knowledge related to Gestalt therapy approach also have a high level of knowledge on diagnostic systems, personality theories, psychopathology, and other therapy approaches. Furthermore, they go through a long-term therapy to be fully aware of themselves as well as to increase their therapeutic skills and experiences, and they are supervised. According to Latner (1986, 146) the Gestalt therapists who complete such a long and dense training are aware of "now" and "here" not only during therapy but also in their daily lives and carry out their life by establishing contacts, by integration, and by accepting their own responsibilities.

PART II:
BASIC CONCEPTS

4

AWARENESS

Awareness is one of the most basic concepts of the Gestalt approach, which considers it as the primary condition of growth and change (Latner 1992). Hence, to develop the skills for awareness and to raise its level are very important goals for therapy.

The Meaning of Awareness

The dictionary definition of *awareness* is knowledge or perception of a situation or fact. Perls et al. (1951/1996, 106) define *awareness* as "a person's being in touch with his/her perception field." Clarkson and Mackewn (1993, 44), who elaborated this description a little further, defined *awareness* as "a person's being in touch with his/her sensations, feelings, thoughts, and behavior, that is, with his/her being and environment."

Awareness is an indicator that shows that a person is alive and who and what sort of a person he/she is (Zinker 1990). According to Yontef (1993, 183), awareness is a way of life. David Schiller (1994) in his book *My Little Zen Friend* has expressed this beautifully as "The purpose of life is to live and to live is to be aware." Awareness, in a sense, shows a similarity with the concept of enlightenment from Eastern philosophy. The person who is aware forms a new meaning related to a given situation, object, person, or to him/herself. While Perls et al. (1951/1996, 106) liken awareness to the light produced by burning coal, for Polster and

Polster (1974, 213), it is like the sunlight that illuminates whatever it falls on. Shub (1994a, 4), on the other hand, explains awareness through the metaphor of a volcano preparing to erupt; when pressure increases, hot lava starts to boil and fissures start to appear, lava starts to burst up, smoke covers everywhere, and the temperature of the air, land, and sea changes. In the process of awareness also, the person first starts to perceive certain things; these perceptions eventually become more defined, and the person starts to experience certain things not only cognitively but also with his/her feelings and body and eventually these appear as new knowledge, a new understanding, or a new point of view. Just as the view changes after the eruption of the volcano, a new view is now relevant for the person who has become aware. The person starts to give a different meaning to his/her previous experiences. Just like the lava overheating or burning its environment, some of the things the person has become aware of might lead him/her to be uneasy and unhappy or to feel pain. However, as the person integrates and reorganizes those things he/she has become aware of, he/she sees that there are different alternatives and changes his/her choices; then the new awareness brings joy, variety, excitement, and novelty.

Characteristics of Awareness

a. Awareness Appears in the "Here and Now"

In the Gestalt approach, awareness and the here and now are an inseparable duo. What is meant by here and now is not the determination of what happened in the past and what should happen in the future but defining what is happening at that very moment. Awareness appears only in the here and now (Perls 1973, 63). Hence, during therapy, the client is asked to fully focus on the existing moment. During the session, while the client is talking about a past situation or an expectation, he/she is reliving them at that moment, that is, in the present. Therefore, what he/she has become aware of is related to neither the past nor the future but to the present moment. Actually, as the past is gone and the future has not arrived, there is only one actual time, and that is now (Perls 1969, 61). In other words, the past and the future become meaningful only when seen through the present time. In Gestalt therapy, in order to emphasize the significance of the present, the client is asked to change whatever has been told related to the past or the future into the present tense. For example, when the client says, "When I came home, not finding my mother there used to upset me very much," the therapist asks the client to express this as "I am coming home, and not finding my mother there upsets me very much." In this way, it is possible for the client to experience what he/she is talking about in the therapy room at that moment and to become aware of his/her perceptions, feelings, thoughts, and actions related to what is being experienced. Being aware of this enables the person to see that he/she has different alternatives and to try them out directly.

b. Awareness Appears Due to the Figure-Ground Relation and the Phenomenology of the Person

There is a multitude of things we can be aware of in a certain moment. In the beginning, an object, person, situation, event, feeling, sensation, thought, or the like might not get our attention. All these things create our background at that moment, and eventually, one of them appears as the figure. That is to say, what we are aware of at a certain moment creates the figure and what we are not aware of the ground (Clarkson 1991, 32). The ground has an unlimited potential. What will become the figure at a certain moment and how the figure will be organized and given meaning depends on the phenomenology of that person or, in other words, depends on his/her unique world (Sills et al. 1998, 33). For example, seeing that their father is frowning, one of the brothers who got a bad grade at school that day may interpret this as the father being angry with him, while the other brother who that morning has heard his father having a work-related argument on the phone may interpret it as his father having something on his mind.

Yontef (1993, 184) has emphasized the role of people's needs in defining what is to be recognized and in giving meaning to it. The things that the person is aware of can lead to excitement, energy, and enlightenment only when they relate to the person's needs. Otherwise, that is, if the emerging figure does not lead to excitement, energy, and enlightenment, such awareness has no impact, meaning, or power for that person. For example, when you are walking on the street, you may be aware of a lot of other people walking too, but this awareness has a meaning for you only when you encounter someone you know. Or while talking with someone, if what is being talked about is not a subject that has a meaning for you, your attention starts to wander and you start thinking about other things or paying attention to other people.

c. Awareness Has Different Components

In order to achieve full awareness, a person has to become aware of his/her mental, emotional, and bodily experiences, his/her environment, as well as the relation between his/her internal experiences and the environment. For example, in situations where the person is aware of his/ her thoughts on a certain issue but unaware of the feelings related to it or is aware of what/she is doing but unaware of what others are doing, then full awareness cannot be experienced. Failure to experience full awareness obstructs growth and development. On the other hand, in terms of therapy, what is not recognized, that is, what is not turned into a figure and remains in the ground is just as important as the recognized ones (Shub 1994a, 14). Passons (1975, 45) indicated that lack of awareness is generally related to avoidance, that is, the person is trying to avoid certain things by choosing not to be aware of them.

In order to achieve full awareness, the person has to be aware of the three components called by Perls (1969) inner, outer and middle regions and internal experiences, environmental factors, and reconciliation field in this book.

1. *Awareness of internal experiences.* This means a person's awareness of his/her sensations, behaviors, feelings, wishes, and value judgments (Polster and Polster 1974, 213). Let's look at them closely:

Awareness of Sensations and Behaviors

For many people, it is not at all easy to be aware of sensations. Particularly in our times where intellectual characteristics are overrated and bodily and emotional traits are pushed to the background, being aware of sensations becomes even more difficult. A person's awareness of hunger, thirst, manner of sitting, facial expression, different parts of the body, the pains or tensions in the body, the feeling of pressure in the chest, manner of breathing, and so on are related to sensations. Sensations, that are the feelings that appear in the body, establish a starting point for behavior. For example, a person who notices that he/she is thirsty drinks water, the perspiring person tries to find a cool place, the one with a headache takes a painkiller. Hence, in order to be aware of these behaviors and to give meaning to them, it is necessary to begin with becoming aware of these sensations. However, this is not always easy because the connections between sensations and behaviors are generally very complicated. For example, people do not eat only when they are hungry. Eating can be based on many reasons, such as the arrival of mealtime, because the meal is ready, because there will not be a chance to eat later on, assuming a later hunger, not wanting to eat alone and being in the company of friends, or not to be able to find that particular food anywhere else. On the other hand, those who are on a diet, who have eating disorders, or who are depressed may forego eating even when they are hungry. Hence it is a serious mistake to assume either that he/she is eating because he/she is hungry when we see someone eating or to conclude that he/she is not hungry if a person is not eating.

> *Which of your sensations are you aware of now? Are you hungry? Are you thirsty? What is happening in your body? Are you sitting? How are you sitting? Are you lying down? How is your posture? Do you feel pain, aches, numbness, or tension in any part of your body? How are you breathing?*

Awareness of Feelings

Many people do not give sufficient importance to their feelings and even believe that being emotional is a weakness. The number of people who apply for therapy complaining, "I am very emotional and I want to get over it," is quite considerable. Actually, the problem is not being emotional or being aware of one's emotions but an inability to express feelings or to find the connections between emotions, sensations, thoughts, and behavior or to integrate these within oneself and the environment. People who are not aware of their feelings face great difficulties in their relationships, and what is more are not aware of why they are having these difficulties. Such people generally answer the question, "What are you feeling?" by telling you what they are thinking. For example, Margaret one day started the session by talking about her relationship with one of her friends and how that friend had given her very curt answers that day. When asked how this made her feel, her response was "I felt that she was resentful toward me," whereas her friend's being resentful toward her is not a feeling but a thought. When Margaret was asked what she felt when she thought that her friend was resentful, her answer was "I felt that she was jealous of me." In this answer, even though Margaret mentioned a feeling, it is a feeling that does not belong to her but to her friend, which means that Margaret still did not express her own feeling. As the exploration continued, Margaret became aware of how angry she was with her friend because of the curt answers she gave. As can be seen in this case, for some people, being aware of their feelings can be very difficult. On the other hand, some people are aware of only some of their feelings and blind to others. For example, men are generally more aware of their anger and women of their sadness.

> *What are you feeling just now? Are you aware of a specific feeling such as joy, excitement, sadness, anger, or some other feeling? Which of your feelings are you more easily aware of? Which feelings do you avoid recognizing? Which feelings are you afraid of other people expressing? Which of their feelings do you judge?*

Awareness of Wishes

Knowing what we want enables us to plan and mobilize to attain it, and achieving our wishes makes us feel happy and self-assured. However, to be aware of what one wants is not easy for many people. Particularly for those who were raised in families where their wishes and needs were not attended to, being aware of them is even harder. Also, as everything seems unimportant and meaningless to people with depression, they may not even desire anything. However, people who have no wishes have no future either. Wishes not only bind the present and future together, they also summarize the past. In some cases, for example, to come across a friend while walking on the street can make you happy, even though you had not previously wished or planned for this. However, constantly not knowing what one wants, leaving everything to coincidences and to the flow of things lead to monotony and loss of joy. Those who are not aware of their wishes either do not achieve anything because they cannot mobilize or cannot get satisfaction from what they have achieved coincidentally. When such people are asked about what they want, they give very general responses, such as "I want to be happy," "I want attention," or "I want to have fun." Unless these wishes are defined exactly, for example, unless what being happy, receiving attention, and having fun means for that person is clear and explained with examples, it is not possible to determine how these wishes are to be met.

> *What are your wishes these days? What are the things you wanted before but do not want now? What are you doing to attain your wishes? How are you preventing yourself from doing this?*

Awareness of Value Judgments

This covers a larger field than being aware of sensations, feelings, and wishes. Even if people are more aware of certain value judgments, they are unaware of many others. From time to time, all of us may say one thing but actually do another. For example, there are many people who say that sex is quite natural but cannot live out their sexuality in a natural and relaxed way. Again, some others despite saying "Of course we are humans, we can make mistakes" have no tolerance even for their smallest mistakes, and judge themselves.

> *What are your value judgments regarding sex or making mistakes? Are there any subjects where you think one way and act in another? For example, what are your value judgments regarding women, men, children and the elderly?*

2. *Awareness of environmental factors.* In order to be aware of environmental factors, it is necessary primarily to be in contact with the environment, which can be achieved with the functional use of the sense organs, that is, by seeing, hearing,

smelling, tasting, and touching. In terms of achieving contact with the environment, development of speaking and movement skills is also important.

What are you aware of regarding your environment just now? Listen to the sounds or the silence around you. How does the place you are in smell? What is the thing you are sitting or lying on made of? Is it soft? Is it comfortable? What are the furnishings around you? Are you aware of their colors? Are there any other people around you? If there are, are you aware of what they are doing, what they are feeling?

3. *Awareness of the reconciliation* field. The most important characteristic of the reconciliation field is the fact that it brings together internal experiences and environmental factors. This field, as can be understood from its name, provides accord and harmony between internal experiences and environmental factors. The awareness related to inner experiences and environmental factors is cognitively organized and given a meaning in this field. Thoughts, dreams, memories, and expectations are located here, and prediction, planning, creation, and making choices are also included in the reconciliation field. Consequently, the reconciliation field is an area that, while causing a lot of problems, when a good harmony is achieved, can also make life richer, more creative, and more enjoyable.

Right now, sit quietly and try to be aware of the thoughts, memories, fantasies, and expectations passing through your mind. Do not focus or dwell too much on any of them. Just be aware of one and pass on to the next. After going on like this for a while, choose an incident you have experienced today and start thinking about it. How do you interpret this incident? What does it mean to you? Did that incident evolve as you wanted it to? If not, what could you have done to make it different?

It is expected that a healthy person will be aware of his/her inner experiences and environmental factors in an equal degree and will consider both of these in his/her evaluations within the field of reconciliation. However, as some people are more aware of their inner experiences and others of the environmental factors, they are unable to experience full awareness in the reconciliation field. For example, thirty-four-year-old Sue came for therapy with complaints such as listlessness, tiredness, and inability to enjoy life. She was successful in her job, but lately, her work performance had been declining, and she was going to work very unwillingly. She was living with her mother and not going out, including the weekends, unless necessary. She no longer knew what she liked to do or what would be good for her; and when she was with others, as she had no preferences of her own, left the decisions of what to do and where to go to them and was even letting her mother choose her outfits. It is apparent from these that Sue's level of awareness of her inner experiences was extremely low. Bruce, on the other hand, applied for therapy because of problems with his wife. He could not spare any time for her or their children because he was spending the time outside his work on exercising, watching television, or reading the newspaper. He was extremely involved with his body and the muscle pains or headaches he had from time to time made him panic, ending in rushed visits to the doctor each time, and in detailed tests. As can be seen, Bruce's level of awareness regarding environmental factors such as his relations with his wife and children in particular and with the other persons around was very low. Emily was going around in a state of perpetual anxiety and was unable to sleep at night as she kept thinking about what others did or said, going over it repeatedly. She was having fits of extreme anger and feeling terribly guilty about them afterwards she was closing herself in. As can be understood, Emily's level of awareness of her field of reconciliation was rather low. She was unable to make her body, feelings, senses, behaviors, and wishes compatible with environmental demands and conditions, to recognize the alternatives and to make appropriate choices.

d. Awareness Is a Dimension

Awareness is a dimension: at one end of it are situations such as being aware of nothing (as in a coma) or being aware of only a very few things (such as sleeping). In either situation, our body carries out its crucial functions. However, unlike the person who is in a coma, the sleeping one is ready to wake up if a potential danger appears. Nevertheless, while sleeping, awareness is at a very low level and automatic. At the other end of this dimension is full awareness. It may be called peak experience or full contact (Joyce and Sills 2003, 27). Contemporary Gestalt therapists such as Fodor (1998) and Resnick (1995, 27) call this peak experience or contact located at the extreme end of the awareness dimension "to be aware that one is aware" or "awareness of awareness." The person who is aware of the things he/she is aware of has an "aha" experience, which is a discovery (Latner 1986, 55). The person being aware of his/her awareness, puts together whatever he/she is aware of through the "aha" experience and organizes them in a new order and, by integrating them, experiences total enlightenment on a specific subject. Expressions such as "I didn't know I was this angry with him," "I didn't realize before that I was the one actually doing the mistreating." "I wasn't aware that for me my work meant being loved" can be given as examples of "aha" experiences. The concept of being aware of being aware has three components such as owning, responsibility, and choice. This means that the person who is aware of his/her awareness can first of all own to what he/she is aware of, that is, his/her sensations, feelings, behaviors, wishes, and needs without criticizing or judging them, can take responsibility for what and how he/she is doing, and based on this, can see that he/she has alternatives in terms of thinking, feeling, and behaving, can choose the ones that are appropriate and can use them.

At this stage, the person feels him/herself vigorous, natural, free, and attached to life and can experience the present moment.

e. Awareness Is the Prerequisite of Mobilization

Awareness is the second phase of the need-satisfaction cycle. It is one of the cornerstones of the Gestalt approach and is located between the sensation and mobilization phases. The healthy person, once aware of a need, mobilizes to satisfy that need by taking into consideration the environmental conditions and his/her alternatives. For example, a person who is feeling lonely, looks over alternatives, such as calling a friend, going to the movies, watching television, reading or exercising and considering the environmental conditions (such as time, money, and weather), starts to actualize one of these alternatives. The stronger and more urgent the matter for awareness is, such as a fire alarm, the clearer and more immediate the mobilization is (Clarkson 1991, 32). On the other hand, being aware of and satisfying some needs can take longer. If a person is to be aware of his/her needs, then he/she has to be aware of the sensations, feelings, thoughts, and behaviors that are at the base of these needs.

How to Work with Awareness in Therapy

Before going into therapy work for raising awareness, it will be worthwhile to look at the criticisms directed by some other therapy approaches to the Gestalt approach because of its emphasis on awareness. According to these critics, the Gestalt approach is overfocused on awareness—that is, consciousness (Polster and Polster 1974, 207). People who come to therapy are already exceedingly aware of everything. Hence, what they really want is not to be aware but to be spontaneous. This criticism might seem valid at first glance, but it should be kept in mind that these people are only aware of what they want to be aware of. For example, a person who washes his/her hands all the time or avoids touching certain things because he/she is scared of catching germs has focused all his/her attention on his/her behavior but has little or almost no awareness of his/her senses, feelings, and other needs. Similarly, a person with difficulty in his/her interpersonal relationships though aware of his/her feelings, thoughts, behaviors, and needs is not fully aware of others or environmental conditions. While the person seems to be protecting him/herself from to be frightened, to worry and to take responsibility, actually what he/she is refusing to be aware of causes various difficulties, and these are what bring him/her to therapy. Hence, according to the Gestalt approach, unless the client is not aware of what he/she is not aware of, it is not possible to leave such difficulties behind.

Another criticism of the Gestalt approach is the claim that so much focus on awareness disrupts the therapy process (Polster and Polster 1974, 209). They explain this with reference to Anderson's famous centipede tale, as follows: Just like the centipede, when asked which of his legs he moves first, started to stumble when he tried to figure it out, the client asked to be aware all the time will not be able to behave spontaneously. However, this criticism fails to take these two points into consideration: First, there is no doubt that for the centipede that has no trouble in walking, being aware of which foot is used when starting to walk might not be important, but those who come for therapy are people who have a problem and thus who are unable to "walk" spontaneously. Therefore, they first of all need to be aware of how they are walking and what the things which obstruct their walking are. Just like a cook who, when a dish lacks flavor, in order to find the cause tries to find out what spoiled its taste by going through the ingredients and how it was cooked, a person who is not satisfied with the taste of life needs to recognize what is spoiling it. Secondly, those who come for therapy may not be aware not only of what is obstructing them from walking spontaneously but also of what should be done and how to ensure that spontaneous walk. Just like a person who has great difficulty in walking after being bedridden for a long time because of an operation, or illness, has to take each step carefully, the client also has to be aware of his/her steps moment by moment for a while before starting to walk easily. Only then will it be possible to walk spontaneously and safely.

Being aware is a life-long process, and one goes through phases of minimum awareness, general or daily awareness, specific awareness experienced from moment to moment, continuing awareness in consecutive moments, and highly developed awareness (Shub 1994a, 8). Since there are always new needs, feelings, thoughts, and experiences emerging in a person's life, awareness should also be continuously renewed and developed. Thus, the Gestalt approach offers a wealth of resources not only for those who have serious psychological problems but for everybody who wants to raise their awareness to develop, grow, and integrate him/herself.

As mentioned previously, in order for a person to meet his/her needs in a healthy manner, first of all he/she has to be aware of his/her self, the environment, and the relations between him/her and the environment. Therefore the goal of awareness work in therapy is to enable the client to gain the skill to be aware of these things and the ability to sustain this awareness. In order to experience full awareness, it is not sufficient to have momentary and sectional awareness of what one is experiencing. Polster (1995, 204) calls such momentary and sectional awareness "vertical." For example, a person's awareness of pressure in the chest at that moment or of feeling sad is momentary and sectional awareness, and unless the person can find the connections between this noticed sense or feeling and his/her needs, impasses, resistances, and styles of contact, that is, if the recognized pressure in the chest or the feeling of sadness remain as isolated experiences, then they cannot contribute to growth and development. Momentary or sectional awareness corresponds to the "insight" concept of other therapy approaches. Burley (1999) explains the stages of momentary or sectional awareness in therapy as follows:

First stage. In this stage, there is an understanding on a mental level. That is, the person understands a certain sense, feeling, behavior, need, or contact style on a mental level and gains insight. For example, a client who is at this stage could recognize on an intellectual level that he/she very much fears being criticized and, because of this, avoids expressing him/herself and eventually feels lonely. However, such awareness, despite enabling the person to understand what he/she is doing intellectually, does not play a significant role in changing his/her ways of behaving. In this stage, the person may have understood what he/she should not do but is not yet aware of what he/she is going to change and how to change it.

Second stage. In this stage, observations related to the situations that are understood intellectually become apparent. For example, a client in this stage could mention such an observation: "I met with my old high-school friends yesterday. I love them very much, and I feel comfortable when I am with them. But yesterday, when we were together, I got very bored and felt lonely because they kept talking about their boyfriends. I didn't have a boyfriend I could talk about." At this stage, the client can observe him/herself better but cannot yet take the responsibility for his/her behavior.

Third stage. In this stage, the client starts to take the responsibility for his/her behavior, starts to bring out more examples and to use expressions such as "I notice/noticed," and "I realize that/ I have realized that." For example, a client at this stage can give examples such as "The other day I was late for a dinner given for a retiring colleague so I had to sit at the very end of the table. When I realized that I was not able to see many people because of my seat, I got very upset. Later I noticed that since I was upset, I couldn't even participate in the conversation of those sitting near me." Such awarenesses show that the client is coming a little closer to change, but it is still too early because the person is not yet aware of how he/she can actually change.

Fourth stage. In this stage, the person starts to be aware of not only what he/she is doing but his/her sensations, feelings, and body. For example, a client could talk in this stage about an event he/she has attended like this: "It was a very crowded meeting and all the relatives had come together. I realized that I was again sitting in a secluded corner of the room and also felt that my stomach was clenching. I was aware that I was wrapping my arms tightly around myself. When I looked at what I was feeling, I realized that I was particularly annoyed with my cousin—my uncle's daughter—because she was sitting at my side in such a way that I couldn't see anybody properly. When I realized this, I moved my chair a little forward and started to sit in a more comfortable position to ease my stomach. As I was still annoyed with my cousin, I didn't talk much, either with her or the others, but I did not feel as alone as before." The awarenesses at this point show that the person has started to understand him/herself better and is much closer to change, but even though the person feels "a little better, a little more comfortable, a little less worried," he/she is not yet sure about what to do and how to do it.

Fifth stage. This is the stage where full awareness has been achieved. Most Gestalt therapists define this phase as "knowing within." In this stage feeling, thoughts, memories, experiences, and fantasies are owned and accepted as they are. For example, the client at this stage could tell his/her story like this: "I once more met my high-school friends and they again started to talk about their boyfriends. Since I didn't have a boyfriend, I had nothing to tell, but this time, instead of sitting there bored, I tried to listen to their problems, thinking that maybe someday it could also happen to me. I realized that I was not as bored as the last time." Even though this is the stage most close to change, one should not expect everything to change at once. Perls (1973) stated that the awareness including sensation, feeling, and understanding is important in terms of growth, but achieving awareness alone is a slow process of development (referred to in Clarkson and Mackewn 1993, 97). Complete change requires the integration of the gained awarenesses within the personality, evaluation of personal and environmental alternatives, and their testing in daily life.

The first step that may be taken in therapy regarding the integration of the attained awarenesses within the personality is to become aware of *sensations*. For this purpose, the therapist asks the client questions such as "What is happening in your body just now?" "Are you aware of how you are breathing at this moment?" "How are you sitting just now?" or "What are you not aware of about your body right now?" In this way, the client may become aware of how, for example, his/her hands feel numb, his/her voice becomes high pitched, and his/her breathing becomes more rapid when he/she is talking about his/her mother. Another subject to be dealt with during awareness work is to become aware of *feelings* and to find out the connections between them and sensations. To that end, the therapist helps the client with questions such as "What are you feeling just now?" "What are you trying not to feel just now?" "What do you feel when your voice becomes high pitched?" or "When your hands become numb at this moment, what are you feeling?" During this work, the client may become aware that, for example, the numbness of the hands is connected to his/her efforts not to feel anything, especially his/her sadness or anger, that his/her queasy stomach is related to his/her fear, or the pressure felt in his/her chest to his/her anxiety. Another subject to be worked on in therapy is awareness of *thoughts* and to investigate the connections between the thoughts, sensations and feelings. For many people, awareness of one's thoughts seems easier, but to see the connections between thoughts, sensations, and feelings is not easy at all. During this work, the client's value judgments are also considered. The therapist makes use of questions such as "What are you thinking just now?" "What is going through your mind?" "What are you trying not to think just now?" "What are you thinking when your hands are numb and your voice is high pitched?" or "What are you thinking when trying not to feel anything?" For example, while the client is answering these questions, he/she can become aware of the fact that while his/her hands are numb and his/her voice high pitched and while he/she is trying not to feel anything at all, his/her thoughts are "I should not be getting angry with my mother. If I become angry, this will be a sin, and I do not want to be unfair to my mother." During therapy, to become aware of *behaviors* and to find out their connection with sensations, feelings, and thoughts is another area that should be worked on. The therapist tries to raise the client's awareness with the help of questions such as "How are you behaving just now?" "How do you behave when you don't want to be unfair to your mother?" or "What are you not saying when your voice becomes high pitched and your breathing accelerates?" It is obvious that awareness work carried out during therapy does not always follow this order. Finding the connections between the sensations, feelings, thoughts, and behaviors is attempted sometimes through behaviors, sometimes through feelings or thoughts.

One other subject that could be taken up during awareness work is the investigation of the connections between the sensations, feelings, thoughts, and behaviors of the person and his/her past. The following is an example of how this could be handled.

Client:	*I don't know what to talk about today.*
Therapist:	*Close your eyes and let yourself go. Tell me what you are aware of, but do not dwell on any of it. Keep letting yourself go.*
Client:	*I am aware of the sound of vehicles outside. I am aware of the slight breeze coming from the window. I am aware that you are sitting over there and looking at me.*
Therapist:	*How does my looking at you make you feel?*
Client:	*Bothers me, having someone looking at me.*
Therapist:	*How does it bother you?*
Client:	*Bad, as if you are observing me.*
Therapist:	*Are you aware of what you are doing with your hand just now?*
Client:	*I noticed when you mentioned it, as if I am petting myself.*
Therapist:	*What are you feeling?*

Client:	*Warmth. I guess I am giving support to myself. I am showing compassion to myself.*
Therapist:	*Keep doing it with your hands. What are you aware of at this moment?*
Client:	*Tears are about to come from my eyes.*
Therapist:	*What are you feeling just now?*
Client:	*Sad.*
Therapist:	*What is making you sad?*
Client:	*I remembered that I was often sick when I was a child. While doctors examined me and observed my body, I used to be ashamed because I grew up rather late. I was very short for years.*

At the later stages of this awareness work, the client became aware of how the negligent attitude of his/her parents toward this late development made her sad and angry, how her negative feelings about her body still caused feelings of shame, and how she was trying to make it invisible.

In the Gestalt approach, the ultimate goal of awareness work is to make the person aware of his/her body, desires, and needs; the ways he/she uses to obstruct the satisfaction of his/her needs; the styles of contact he/she uses; his/her unfinished business, impasses and polarities, and the phase in which he/she is interrupted in the need-satisfaction cycle. Possible work on these aspects that could be utilized in therapy is given in detail in the coming sections.

In conclusion, the skill of awareness can only be learned by experiencing it, and this learning continues throughout life with new awareness. New experiences, developments, and relationships change what is to be recognized and require their continuous renewal. In therapy, the client's attainment of the skill to be aware is very important but not sufficient for growth and change. In order to achieve this, the client should be able to integrate whatever he/she is aware of, to develop new alternatives, to gain the strength for self-support, and to be able to take on his/her own responsibilities.

5

NEEDS

According to the Gestalt approach, the basis of life is needs and its goal is their satisfaction (Serok 2000, 7). Every person has a multitude of needs—physical, social, and spiritual, among others. While some of these are common ones shared by all, some are unique to a particular person. For example, needs such as food, water, sleep, love and attention, appreciation, self-expression, learning, success, and self-protection are common, seen in everybody. However, activities such as engaging in sports, playing a musical instrument, reading books, or writing poetry are very important for some us and are not even considered as a need by others.

Humans have the natural tendency to recognize their needs and to regulate themselves so as to be able to meet them (Mackewn 1999, 17). They can organize their experiences and energy according to their needs by using their physical, cognitive, and emotional capacities in interactions with their environment. The more needs are satisfied in the shortest time with greatest ease, the more comfortable and happy the person will be. Some needs are met in a short time. Satisfaction of certain other needs, such as learning something or establishing a close relationship with someone, requires more time and effort. When the satisfaction of the need takes a long time or is hard, then the balance between the organism and the environment remains disrupted for that longer period. Unmet needs constantly pressure a person and cause unhappiness and distress.

In Gestalt theory, the emergence, priority, and satisfaction of needs are explained through "figure and ground" relations (Clarkson 1991, 5).

Figure and Ground Relations

The figure-ground relation is one of the field theory postulates that are at the root of the Gestalt approach. Field theory was put forward by the German psychologist Kurt Lewin (1952) and is built upon Gestalt perception studies carried out by psychologists such as Wertheimer, Köhler, and Koffka. According to the field theory, during perception and meaning-giving, while some characteristics move to the foreground, some others remain in the background. While the ones in the foreground form the "figure," the ones that are left back form the "ground" (Köhler 1947/1992, 252). During perception, the figure and the ground continuously change places, and what is to be the figure and what the ground may differ from person to person and from one time to another.

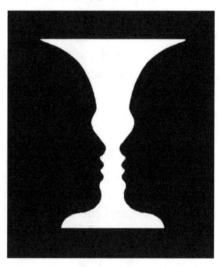

A vase and two people facing each other

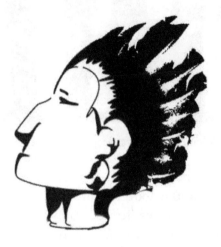

Eskimo and an Indian bust

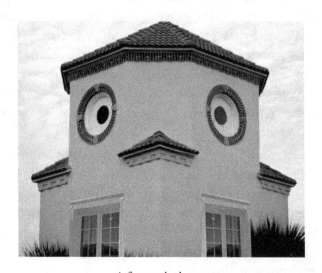

A face and a house

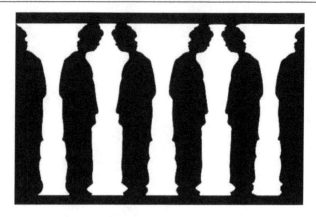

Columns and several people facing each other

For a better understanding of figure-ground relations, it is worthwhile examining the above pictures. When you look at the first picture, if you focus on the white area, you will see a vase; while if you focus on the black area, what you see will be the profiles of two people facing each other. In other words, for those who see the vase in this picture, the black area is the ground, and for those who see two people facing each other, the ground is the white area. In the second picture, there is both a rear view of an Eskimo and an Indian bust. The third picture includes both a face and a house, the fourth columns and several people facing each other. Were you able to see the different figures in the pictures? As you must have noticed, in order to see the different figures, one has to define different areas as the ground, and as the ground changes, figures also change.

During perception, what will move forward and become the figure and what will remain in the back and become the ground is determined according to the needs of the person and his/her level of awareness of these needs. There are many needs in the ground that wait to be satisfied. For a need to become obvious, that is, to become the figure, there should be a stimulus forging change either within the organism or in the environment (Estrup 2000). For example, for the need to eat to emerge, the person either has to be aware of some bodily sensations (such as hunger, stomach spasms, or bowel movements) or has to become aware of environmental factors (such as the smell or sight of food or the arrival of mealtime). In this way, the need to eat, which has so far been part of the ground, becomes the figure and the person acts to satisfy it. When this has been done, that is, when the person is full, this need loses its importance and returns to the ground, remaining there until the person is once again hungry. In the meanwhile, through internal or external stimuli, some other need starts to emerge as the figure. Just now you could be aware of your dry mouth and difficulty in swallowing and thinking that you need to drink something. The moment you think this, the need to read this book has moved to the ground, and the need for a drink of water has become the figure. After quenching your thirst, if you remember that you have to call a friend, then both the need to read this book and to drink something moves to the ground and the need to call your friend is now the figure.

According to the field theory, when a need becomes the figure, tension arises (Rummel 2004). As long as the need is not met, this tension continues, and the longer satisfaction takes, the stronger the tension becomes. A person who becomes aware of a need attempts to mobilize to meet it and starts to set targets, which may have both an attractive (that is, positive) value for the person, as well as irritating (negative) ones. Targets with a positive value make need satisfaction easier and faster, while the negative ones make it harder and slower. Let us assume that, believing that in order to be healthy and fit you have to exercise regularly, you have joined a gym. In such a case, the facilities of the gym, the machines you will be using there and the feeling of self-admiration when you are healthy and fit can encourage you to go to the gym. On the other hand, factors such as the long distance to the facility, hot, cold or rainy weather, your actual dislike of working out on the machines or feeling tired may be negative values that prevent you from going. Ultimately, whether or not you will be exercising regularly—that is to say how the conflict between the positive and negative values will be resolved—is determined by the strength of the basic need. If your need to remain healthy and fit is very strong, you will continue to exercise regularly; if not, you might even forget your gym membership as time passes.

Depending on the field theory, Perls (1973, 19) talked about the concept of positive and negative catharsis. Objects that meet the needs of the people and help in dissolving conflict lead to positive catharsis. For example, water for a thirsty person and a comfortable bed for a tired soul are objects of positive catharsis. Objects that do not meet the needs of a person, which do not contribute to the resolution of the conflict and which threaten the person cause negative catharsis. For example, a barking dog for someone who is scared of them and books for a person who does not like to read are objects of negative catharsis. Naturally, while a person wants to reach those objects, situations, and people in his/her environment that are sources of positive catharsis, he/she will try to stay away from those that create negative catharsis and, if possible, to destroy them. For example, we avoid people who distress us or try to erase bad feelings from our minds. Hence, objects, situations, and people who cause positive and negative catharsis either attract or repel a person like a magnet. There is a mathematical relation between people's needs and catharsis-creating objects (Perls 1973, 22). If the need is due to a lack of something, that is if it is negative (–) (such as being thirsty), then the object leading to catharsis, (water) is positive (+). If the need is born of an excess of something, if it is positive (+) (such as being in a very noisy place), the object causing catharsis, (getting away from the noise) is negative (–). As a result, the sum of the catharsis-causing object and the need will be zero. Hence, when the need that is satisfied through positive or negative catharsis comes to point 0 and disappears; than the tension of the organism comes to an end.

The Need-Satisfaction Cycle

According to the Gestalt approach, when a need emerges, a Gestalt starts to be formed and is completed and closed when the need is satisfied. The Gestalt is destroyed the moment a new need occurs and is completed by the formation of a new Gestalt. The destruction, formation, and completion of the Gestalt proceeds within a cycle, and Perls (1947/1992, 43) named this cycle that related to need satisfaction the "cycle of the inter-dependency of organism and environment." In later years, the cycle was given different names such as the "awareness- excitement-contact cycle" (Zinker 1997, 97), "the cycle of gestalt formation and destruction" (Clarkson 1991, 29), the "experience cycle" (Sills et al. 1998, 48), the "Gestalt experience cycle" (Korb et al. 1989, 25), and the "contact cycle" (Philippson 2001, 42). The cycle can be illustrated as either a circle or a wave.

Perls (1947/1992, 43) defined the following phases in the cycle:

1. The organism is at rest.
2. An internal or external disturbing stimulus emerges.
3. An image is created or a real situation is recognized.
4. A response is given to this.
5. Tension is lowered.
6. The organism returns to a state of balance.

Just like the names given to the cycle, the names of the phases included in the cycle also vary. For example, Sills et al. (1998, 52) call these phases "sensation, recognition, appraisal and planning, action, contact, assimilation and completion, and withdrawal." Clarkson (1991, 29) took up the phases of the cycle in greater detail and named them sensation, awareness of the emergence of a biological or social need, the mobilization and excitement phase of contact, choosing and implementation of the appropriate action, a full and vibrant contact, satisfaction and Gestalt completion, and withdrawal or rest of the organism. Zinker (1977, 97) referred to the phases of the cycle as sensation, awareness, mobilization of energy, action, contact, and withdrawal. Korb et al. (1989, 25), diverging from others, defined eight phases in the cycle and named them rest, need emergence, scan, choice, contact, assimilation or rejection, satisfaction, and withdrawal. In this book, a seven-phase model is used, and the cycle is called the "need-satisfaction cycle." The phases are named as sensation, awareness, mobilization, action, contact, satisfaction and withdrawal. The cycle, illustrated as a wave, is presented below.

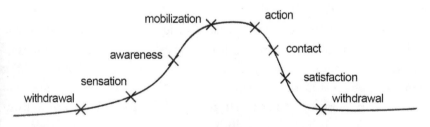

The need-satisfaction cycle shown as a wave

As indicated above, according to this model, in order to satisfy the need, first the person has to be aware of the sensations coming from his/her body or from the environment. For example, while you are reading this book, you might hear a sound (sense), recognize it as the ringing of the telephone (awareness), decide to answer it and reach for the phone (mobilization), answer it and start talking (action). While you are talking (contact), if you can share with the other person whatever you like, you will be very pleased (satisfaction), and put down the phone (withdrawal). Afterward you might start to read this book again to satisfy your unfinished need to read it. In this case, the need to read this book was held up in the contact phase of the cycle during the phone conversation, but this is remedied as soon as you start reading once more. Later, when you have read as much as you want, you stop reading and thus your need to read has been met and the cycle is completed. Likewise, in our daily lives, we satisfy our needs by completing a great number of cycles. Some are short term and completed without pressuring us. Others, such as learning to drive, finishing school, or making a good friend are long term ones. Yet other cycles, such as actualization of oneself, are life-long affairs.

There is no doubt that the meeting of certain needs is not always easy and a person can be interrupted at different phases of this cycle and fail to satisfy those needs. For example, let us assume that after stopping reading, you remember that you had previously arranged to meet with a friend (sensation); when you see the time, you realize that the arranged time was close (awareness), and you start to get ready. You leave to meet him/her (mobilization) and reach your destination thinking about what you were talking about the last time you were together (action). When you reach the meeting place, you wait for a long time, but your friend does not come, that is, you don't meet. In such a situation, this experience is interrupted at the "contact" phase. Or, let us assume that when you arrive at the meeting venue, you find your friend waiting for you. Your friend is very happy to see you, and you sit together and start talking (contact), but just as the conversation is getting into full swing and you are both enjoying it, you see that another friend you both know from way back but you don't like at all is approaching your table. When you realize that she was invited by your friend and she is going to join you, you decide to leave, and feeling very angry with your friend for inviting this person you dislike and for not warning you about this invitation beforehand, you leave shortly. In this situation, as you were unable to talk with your friend as you had wished to, your need was interrupted at the "satisfaction" stage.

In the following pages, the characteristics of each phase and certain problems that could emerge due to interruptions at those phases are discussed.

The Sensation Phase

During the sensation phase, with the appearance of stimuli related to internal or environmental experiences, one of the physical, psychological, or social needs starts to become the figure. The internal stimuli of the person could be physical symptoms such as hunger pains, a dry mouth, or a headache, or they could also be mental stimuli such as thinking about someone or remembering some unfinished business (Korb et al. 1989, 24). Similarly, environmental stimuli can have physical characteristics such as changes in temperature, an earthquake, a sound or a smell, while they can also be related to the people in the environment, such as coming across someone or hearing something from a person. The nonemergence of any internal or environmental sensations can only be possible if the person is under the influence of sedatives, in a coma, in a deep sleep, or in a hypnotic trance. Other than such cases, every person is open to internal or environmental stimuli in varying degrees.

People who are interrupted at the sensation phase or, who have difficulty in passing this phase, cannot distinguish their bodily sensations and are not aware of what they want. It is as if their feelings are frozen, and their emotions have disappeared. In extreme cases, self-harming attempts such as cutting oneself or suicide can be seen. Depressive and nondifferentiated schizophrenic symptoms are due to difficulties experienced at this phase (Zinker 1977, 98). In some cases, serious problems can be faced regarding personal hygiene. While working with those who have difficulties in the sensation phase, the therapist aims at enabling the client to gain awareness of him/herself and his/her environment. The methods that can be used in this regard are taken up in the section on desensitization.

Another problem encountered in this phase is being overly aware of sensations. In such cases, the person is continuously involved with his/

her body and is overly interested in every signal from it. Such people have very low pain thresholds. Constantly watching themselves, they may go through unnecessary checkups or frequently rush to the emergency room in a panic. Another problem seen in the sensation phase is the case where the person is affected by every stimulus from the environment and his/her inability to distinguish those to be taken into consideration from those to be ignored. These people have very poor concentration and have great difficulty in focusing on a specific issue. Those who constantly think about something but are not aware of what it is they are thinking about also have problems at this phase. While working with such clients, the therapist does not help the client to be aware of his/her sensations or the environmental stimuli but, on the contrary, helps the client concerning how he/she can ignore some stimuli, how to slow down, and how to lower his/her energy level.

The Awareness Phase

In this phase, the person starts to be aware of his/her internal sensations or those coming from the environment, to give them meaning, and to distinguish between them. For example, at this phase, the person may become aware of a feeling of pressure in his/her chest and may interpret this as catching a cold and about to become sick. For another person, this pressure could be a hint of how sad he/she is. A person hearing an alarm from the street can tell whether it belongs to his/her car or to someone else's. Sometimes a person becomes aware of a past memory or an expectation regarding the future (Yontef and Simkin 1989).

People who have problems during the awareness phase are aware of their sensations but have serious difficulties in naming them and giving them a meaning. Consequently, they cannot be aware of their needs. When a person with difficulties at this stage comes for therapy, he/she is aware of the fact that something is just not right, but he/she is not clear about what is going wrong. Such people also find their bodily stimulants weird and even scary and evaluate them either incompletely or in a wrong way. For example, a person having difficulties in this phase, despite not experiencing any other symptoms, may judge the increased heart rate and rapid breathing as a heart attack and not even consider that these symptoms might be a sign of anxiety. These incomplete and mistaken evaluations also often emerge in psychosis. For example, a person who feels numbness in his/her head may give this a meaning as if actually millions of ants are moving around in his/her head and eating his/her brain. Another person may interpret the police car seen on the street as meaning that the police are coming to catch him/her, despite the fact that no crime has been committed. Some other people who have blockages in the awareness phase may be overly impulsive and energetic. As they cannot give meaning to the internal and environmental sensations they are fully aware of, they can act without thinking, suddenly and impulsively. People with passive- aggressive personality characteristics are also among those who have difficulties at this phase. While working with such clients, the goal of the therapist is to help the client to give correct and realistic meanings to the internal and environmental sensations he/she is aware of. The methods that may be used to that end are discussed in the sections on awareness, body language, and deflection.

The Mobilization Phase

In the mobilization phase, the person has determined what the need is and started to think about, investigate, and plan his/her available alternatives to satisfy it. In a sense, during this phase of the cycle, the person is involved in evaluating the situation and, then having decided what to do to, will be ready to mobilize. However, people who experience a blockage at this stage, despite knowing what their needs are and the alternative means of satisfying them, cannot mobilize. When such people come for therapy, they complain about constant procrastination and laziness. For example, they use expressions such as "I know I have to study, but I just can't get into it," or "I want to call my friends, but I just can't pick up the phone." One of the most frequently encountered symptoms in this phase is indecision, whose basic cause is the fear and anxiety these people are experiencing regarding need- satisfaction instead of enthusiasm and excitement. Fear and anxiety lead to the blockage of their energy and most obviously affect the manner of breathing. Because of this, the breathing of psychotics and neurotics is very shallow (Zinker 1977, 102). This type of breathing affects in particular the recognition and expression of feelings. People with depression and anxiety disorder face very serious problems in this phase, which is also difficult for those with obsessive-compulsive personality characteristics or disorders.

The interventions practiced in terms of this phase during therapy aim to help the client to become aware of at which part of his/her body and how the energy is blocked and to release his/her energy. However, during work carried out to overcome the difficulties experienced in this phase, the initial focus is on making the person aware of and understanding how he/she is interrupting him/herself and how this awareness and understanding is not sufficient for mobilization. In other words, to have the person understand his/her self, family, marriage, or situation only by talking with the therapist or by reading does not mobilize him/her. For this reason, in the Gestalt therapy approach, it is believed that in order for a person to mobilize, beyond understanding the interruptions he/she has used, the person has to experience these ways he/she used to interrupt him/herself in therapy. What prevent a person from mobilizing could sometimes be feelings such as anger, sorrow, or anxiety, sometimes wrong or incomplete information that has been introjected, and sometimes bodily reactions. Hence, during therapy the client is supported in expressing these negative feelings as well as his/her positive feelings such as joy, happiness, pride, and love, not only verbally but also bodily and vocally. The ways to overcome the difficulties encountered in this phase are given in detail in the sections on introjection and resistance.

The Action Phase

In this phase, the person has defined his/her needs, made the necessary plans to meet them, and started to use his/her emerging energy in a goal-oriented manner. Now, cognitive, behavioral, and emotional activities are organized. The person aims to meet his/her needs in the most feasible way by discarding some of the various alternatives and by trying out those that might work. People who are interrupted and face difficulties in the action phase, despite possessing sufficient energy for the realization of their plans, somehow cannot take the appropriate action that will meet their needs and attain their goals. For example, a person who has difficulties at this stage can neither clearly put forward his/her wishes nor ask for help from others or give honest reactions. Somatic symptoms such as tachycardia, high blood pressure, or various muscle pains are frequently seen in such people. Male impotence is also related to difficulties encountered at this phase. Catatonic schizophrenia and psychotic depression are also very serious disturbances related to this phase. Hysterical personality characteristics can also be seen in those who have a hard time at this phase (Zinker 1977, 108).

The goal of therapy at this phase is the elimination of the obstructing causes preventing the person from taking the actions he/she wants to take. Projections depending on unassimilated introjections play a significant role in the interruption of the person's realizing what he/she wants to do. Consequently, while the therapist is working with people who are stuck at this phase, he/she first investigates the person's thoughts, beliefs, and attitudes regarding him/herself, others, and relationships and helps the client in changing and integrating the relevant ones. At this stage, the therapist also asks the client to imagine the acts he/she is afraid of or shy about or to actually do them in the therapy room. The Gestalt approach has many exercises that can be used in terms of the mobilization phase. Some of them are given in the sections on projection and polarities.

The Contact Phase

The person in the contact phase is undertaking the activities, experiencing the relations, and acting as necessary for the realization of his/her goals. This phase is completely practice-oriented. Those who have difficulties at this phase are perpetually in motion. While trying to realize what they want in the best possible fashion, they actually do not establish full contact with what they are doing, seeing, or hearing. Likewise, as they cannot establish full and deep contact with people either, even though there are many people around them, they have no close friends. The same situation is also relevant for those who are frequently changing sex partners. People who have problems in the contact phase cannot properly adjust the distance in their interpersonal relations and have a need for a very frequent and intensive type of contact. They are so afraid of being alone that they always want the company of others. Since they have a tendency not to hear messages coming from others, they cannot determine the balance of give and take in their relations. They cannot understand that other people may not want to be constantly in contact and do not want to allow them to withdraw. Consequently, they are refused and pushed away by others. Another difficulty experienced in this phase is the person's tendency to have no contact at all. For example, a person rejected and pushed away after very frequent and intensive contacts may withdraw completely and could even start not to establish contact at appropriate times and settings. Similarly, an obsessive-compulsive person who is constantly washing his/her hands may after a while become so tired of this washing that he/she could start not to wash his/her hands at all. Again, a person who is greatly hurt during a manic period may stop contacting and go into a depressive period.

During therapy, while working with clients who are experiencing very frequent and intensive contacts, the goal is to help them to focus on the here and now and to be aware of his/her feelings. To that end, the client's habit of constantly being busy with other people or things is prevented and he/she is encouraged to remain silent and immobile and to be aware of his/her own sensations and feelings. Staying silent and immobile leads to the appearance of anxiety, and this causes previously unrecognized problems to surface and only then it is possible to work on these problems. While working with noncontacting, isolated clients, the goal is to help the person to establish and sustain contact. Methods that can be used during therapy regarding the difficulties encountered during the contact phase are given in the sections on body language and retroflection.

The Satisfaction Phase

In this phase, the person has realized his/her goal and consequently experiences full satisfaction both physically and psychologically. The Gestalt is completed; the need is met, what was targeted is achieved. Satisfaction is what a mother feels when she first holds and feeds her baby, what a student feels when receiving his/her diploma, and what a man feels when he completes his military service. The satisfaction stage is the quiet after the storm, the precious moments just before separation or withdrawal begins (Clarkson 1991, 35). In this phase, to reach satisfaction, the need does not necessarily have to be met with objects or people that create positive catharsis. For example, meeting the person's need for spending a nice day with his/her family as well as his/her need for a good cry or to break off a bad relationship can be satisfactory purely by giving a feeling of relief and content. People who face difficulties in the satisfaction phase are those who are never happy with what they have achieved no matter what they do, those who cannot be satisfied until they achieve perfection, and those who always look for what is missing or wrong. Such people do not know how to enjoy what they have or fully digest it. They constantly try to control themselves and those around them. They never let themselves go and feel inadequate. People with narcissistic characteristics are also among those who have difficulties in this phase.

While working with people who have difficulties at the satisfaction phase, the goal is to enable the client to let him/herself go and to give spontaneous and natural reactions. For this, the client is helped to pay attention not on the past or the future but on the existing moment, to not constantly see him/herself through the eyes of others but through his/her own eyes and not to focus on only him/herself or the immediate environment, but on the contact boundary between him/herself and the environment. For interventions that can be used during therapy regarding this phase, the section on egotism could be useful.

The Withdrawal Phase

This phase is both the end and the beginning of the need-satisfaction cycle. Now the need is met, satisfaction achieved, and the satisfied need has once again moved to the ground. The person remains at this phase until a new need emerges. Perls (1976) calls this phase the "infertile void" (referred to in Sills et al. 1998, 52). At this phase, the person is open to all types of sensations, feelings, thoughts, wishes, and environmental stimuli. The withdrawal phase is the prerequisite of the formation of a new gestalt. People who cannot terminate any job, thought, or contact are those who encounter difficulties in this phase. In interpersonal relationships, they are neither aware of their own boundaries nor those of the others. These people are greatly disturbed by being away from someone for any length of time or by breaking off a relationship even if it has been making them unhappy. Those who have difficulties in the withdrawal phase are constantly active and busy with something. Workaholics are one of the best examples of this. While some workaholics complain, some others are satisfied with themselves. However, complaining or not, they continue to be in continuous motion. Moreover, such people do not realize when they are tired or need sleep. Behaviors such as excessive eating or excessive alcohol consumption are also often seen in those who have problems with this phase. Some others who are experiencing an interruption during this phase are constantly uneasy as they keep thinking about the object, situation, person, or job they have not chosen, worrying whether or not they will be sorry later. For these people, it could be very difficult to finish a conversation, to leave when visiting, and even to turn off the television. People with symptoms of obsessive-compulsive behavior also experience difficulties at the withdrawal stage. For example, those with a compulsion for constant hand-washing may not realize how tired they are; even if they are aware, they may ignore it and continue washing. Since they are not focused on what they are doing and the moment they are in, they cannot be sure if they have washed enough and therefore need to wash their hands again and again. Those who compulsively collect also have difficulties in this phase. In extreme cases, such people cannot part with and throw away clothes and possessions that have become obsolete, broken, or unusable, and hold on even to objects such as boxes, shopping bags, and papers. The manic phase of the manic depressive psychosis is a serious disturbance that occurs in connection with this phase.

The goal of the therapy applied to clients who have difficulties in the withdrawal phase is to help them to become aware of the boundaries of the others as well as their own, to gain the strength to protect their boundaries, and to develop the skill of self-support. The exercises that could be used to this end are given in the sections on introjection and confluence.

To sum up, according to the Gestalt approach, in the satisfaction of a need, or in other words, in the formation, completion, and destruction of the Gestalt, it is imperative to go through the phases of sensation, awareness, mobilization, action, contact, satisfaction, and withdrawal. Difficulties encountered in these phases make a person fail to meet his/her needs that in turn cause unhappiness and lead to psychological problems. Should a person get stuck at any one of these phases, then it is impossible for him/her to go on to the next and close the cycle. For example, if the person is stuck at the mobilization phase, he/she cannot move on to the contact, satisfaction, or withdrawal phases before overcoming the difficulties faced at this phase. The need satisfaction cycle is one of the maps utilized while making a diagnosis according to the Gestalt approach. Determination of the phase the person is stuck at through this map is very important in terms of planning the path to be followed in therapy and the techniques to be used. How this map is used is described in the section entitled "A Case Presentation."

Another issue which is important in terms of the path to be followed and the techniques to be used in therapy is knowing the factors that are preventing need satisfaction. These factors are individually discussed in the following pages.

Factors Preventing Need Satisfaction

a. Judgment of Needs

If a need is to be met, first it has to be recognized, that is, it has to become a figure (Simkin and Yontef 1984). The most important factor in not noticing a need is refusing to see it as a need and even to judge it as "what sort of a need that is," to see it as "unnecessary," "ridiculous," or even as "harmful." The primary cause of disowning a need, on the other hand, is the rigid value judgments that have been introjected (Perls et al. 1951/1996, 119). Many of us criticize other people's needs based on information we have introjected without questioning. For example, if being slim is a very important need for us, we criticize those who are overweight and try to prevent their eating, or if reading is very important for us, we might force other people to read and even demean them for not reading. What is more, we do all this "for their own good." However, even if we act with the best of intentions, in the end, we are actually being disrespectful of their needs. Everybody has different needs, and everybody has the right to meet these in a way appropriate for them.

There is no doubt that we not only judge the needs of the others but also judge our own. For example, since some people regard crying as a sign of weakness, even if they are sad about something and want to cry, they make an excessive effort not to cry and show their sorrow.

The repetitive judgment and suppression of the need to cry eventually leads to the person's inability to cry, and in time, it can even prevent the person from noticing his/her feelings of sorrow. Because of this, some people when they feel sorrow reflect it externally as anger. Some people believe that sex is very shameful, ugly, or not necessary, even though it is completely natural. They feel extremely disturbed when faced with internal or external sexual stimuli and, in order not to feel disturbed, close themselves to all such stimuli and become sexually frigid individuals. However, whether fitting the introjected values or not, when a need emerges, it definitely has to be satisfied through appropriate means otherwise it will come out at the most inappropriate moments and in the most unlikely manners (such as crying fits or outbursts of anger) and put one in a difficult spot. Perls et al. (1951/1996, 32) pointed out that giving up one's needs because of the value judgments of others or of society causes a significant loss in a person's energy and will to live.

In some cases, the reason behind judging needs is the fact that the person's needs and those of people in his/her environment are not compatible; that is, there is a conflict between these two sets of needs. People who grow up with messages such as "To do whatever one wants is selfishness," "One should relinquish his/her desires in order not to upset loved ones," "You mustn't go against your parent's wishes," or "You should obey your elders," believe that one of the parties has to give up his/her needs, or they experience serious conflicts by blaming other people or themselves. For example, Paula had a long-term relationship that was going just fine, but her boyfriend had a job that her father hated and was living in another city. Paula's mother, on the other hand, had no intention of sending her daughter away to a different city. Her parents had never actually met the boyfriend, but they were sure that Paula could not be happy with him. However, Paula felt that she would be happy with him and wanted to marry him. Her boyfriend was determined not to give Paula up and wanted to marry her anyway when he graduated from university, even without the consent of her parents. Close to his graduation, Paula realized that she could never convince her parents and told him that she could not marry him. In this way, Paula judged her need for a man she loved and would be happy with, ignored her own needs, and decided that the needs of her parents were more important than her own. However, when later Paula showed symptoms of introversion, inability to enjoy life, and staying in bed all day long, her parents brought her for therapy. Paula's problems were based on her failure to find a balance between her own need to love and be loved, her father's prejudices, her mother's need not to be separated from her, and not to be able to manage the necessary adjustments because of a variety of messages she had introjected.

b. Failure to Prioritize Needs

As previously mentioned, humans have a great variety of needs and these, by becoming figures, constantly put pressure on a person to satisfy them. Hence, the person has to organize his/her hierarchy of needs, taking into consideration his/her own priorities and environmental conditions (Serok 2000, 8). While prioritizing, the person defines his/her needs as he/she perceives them and according to the perceived aspects of the environment (Korb et al. 1989, 7). Consequently, each person's priority of needs is unique. If more than one need emerges at a specific moment, the person should define the most important among them and meet that one first. In this regard, Perls (1951/1996, 277) gives the example of a soldier in the desert. For a thirsty soldier who has stayed in the desert for a long time, water is a very important need, and hence, as soon as he returns to his camp, he goes for water. This soldier has also been waiting for a promotion for a long time. Just as he is going for a drink of water, his commander stops him and tells him that his promotion has come through. However, the soldier is so thirsty that, even though he hears this news, he still goes on to get water, feeling nothing and showing no reaction. Just at that moment, the camp is attacked and the need for drinking water loses its significance for the soldier, and he starts to fight as his need to protect himself and the camp has become prominent. As can be seen in this example, this soldier was able to determine what his most important need was according to the conditions of the moment and was able to rearrange the other needs. However, determination of the most dominant need may not always be so easy and may strain a person. If the person is unable to define what his/her dominant need is at a given moment and tries to satisfy several needs simultaneously, then he/she cannot organize him/herself and his/her environment and act effectively (Perls 1973, 18). The person who cannot satisfy his/her needs effectively eventually feels more and more apathetic and lacks energy (Perls 1951/1996, 275). For example, Patricia, who is twenty-five years old, after successfully finishing school, started to work and thought that her most important need at that time was to succeed in this. She further believed that if she was successful at her job, she would be loved by everybody and thus satisfy through her work her need to be loved. Consequently, she worked very hard and did everything asked of her, and even what was not requested. She tried her best to have her colleagues love her and, from time to time, took on their tasks. With all this, she started to work until increasingly late hours. In a short time, she had become really good at her job, and her success was appreciated by everybody. However, Patricia started to feel lonely, restless, lacking in energy, and started to have problems on concentrating. As she was so very tired and listless by the time she left work, she was too burned out when she got home even to chat with her parents. Meanwhile she could not find the time and the energy to be with her friends. Her family and friends started to reproach her. In order to gain their forgiveness, Patricia bought gifts for them with the money she earned but was aware that this is not pleasing them. On the other hand, Patricia had always enjoyed exercising before but had to give it up because of her job; she started to gain weight as she became sedentary and thus did not like herself physically either. As she felt unhappy and could not find anything to share with her seldom-met friends because of her shrinking field of interests, she did not want to meet them anymore. Meanwhile, since she was always feeling tense and restless, her relationship with her new boyfriend was also suffering. Finally, Patricia, feeling very unhappy, applied for therapy with complaints of irritation, a feeling of emptiness, perpetual tiredness, and apathy as well as muscle and joint pains. As can be seen, at the root of Patricia's complaints lies her sole effort to be successful, her failure to prioritize her other needs (such as establishing close relations, sharing, exercising, having fun) and her failure to make adjustments in this list of priorities from time to time.

c. Unfinished Business

Another factor that plays a role in the failure to satisfy needs is unfinished business. The more unfinished business a person has, the harder the satisfaction of current needs becomes (Serok 2000, 12). One of the best examples that can be given in this regard is a person's inability to meet his/her need for sleep because of unfinished business (Perls et al. 1951/1996, 441–442). It is obvious that everybody needs to sleep and rest every day at certain hours. However, some people or sometimes all of us, despite needing rest and relaxation, suffer from insomnia. This is because, at that time, our real need is not to sleep but to satisfy our yet unfinished need. While there is a need waiting for satisfaction, efforts at going to sleep cause the repression of the real need. Since the person is not aware of which of his/her needs is to be satisfied and how, he/she tries various ways to fall asleep. For example, some people say that they fall asleep while watching television, but they cannot sleep when they move to their beds. Although this type of short-time sleeping helps the body rest for a while, as it does not go on for a sufficient time and as it is not of high quality, it indicates that the mind of the person is full of a multitude of emotional needs experienced all day long but not completed. In cases of chronic insomnia, the unfulfilled need lies much deeper. We generally tend to blame our inability to sleep on environmental conditions. For example, we see the dog barking outside or the noise from our neighbor as the cause of our inability to sleep. Thus we direct our anger at the dog or the neighbor. We could possibly throw something at the barking dog or knock on the ceiling to shut our neighbor up. In this situation, if our unfinished business is related to a feeling of anger, we might experience partial relief, but as we have not fully met our need, we wake up again after a while. In such cases, the most healthy thing, instead of trying to sleep, would be to try to stay awake, to find out what our unfinished business is, to achieve the emotional release we need by verbal expressions, fantasy illustrations, or writing it down and, if necessary, to make an active plan. More information on unfinished business and how it can be dealt with in therapy is given in detail in the section on unfinished business.

d. Anxiety Due to Unstarted Business

Under normal circumstances, when a need becomes clear, energy is released and the person mobilizes to meet the need. The energy emerging for mobilization causes more rapid breathing, an increase in the blood flow to the heart, brain, lungs, and peripheral organs and the mixing of glycogen into the bloodstream. Energy flow manifests itself as vitality, warmth, and brightness, and in the Gestalt approach, this is called "excitement" (Kepner 1987, 137). In other words, excitement is the increase in energy when a need appears. Excitement enables the person to be active, creative, and vivid (Clarkson 1991, 90). However, if the excitement is blocked, then the person starts to feel anxiety, which renders the person passive, immobile, and monotonous. Anxiety is generally experienced in areas such as bereavement, suffering harm, or loss of love or attention, which threaten the physical or psychological well-being of the person (Korb et al. 1989, 15). According to the Gestalt approach, anxiety is a future-oriented feeling. The person who experiences the moment he or she is in feels excitement and acts spontaneously. On the other hand, pondering the future causes a person to go into catastrophic or anastropic expectations. Anastropic expectations, which are positive, enable the person to mobilize immediately to meet his/her needs. Catastrophic expectations, on the other hand, concern negative and bad things that may happen and, by blocking a creative release of energy, cause the energy to move toward obsessive thinking or unrealistic activities (Korb et al. 1989, 54).

Another factor that plays a role in the failure to meet needs is having extreme expectations and trying to arrange one's life according to them (Serok, 2000, 13). Everyone has a lot of fantasies, dreams, and expectations; however, as some people have a need to control the future, they keep calculating the possibilities of realizing these fantasies, dreams, and expectations and thus cannot mobilize. These people have a tendency to constantly postpone the future. They prevent the satisfaction of their needs through a timescale of procrastination: "Later," "When I am retired," "When the children grow up," or "When the schools are on holiday"; thus they cannot start anything new. The expectations and anxieties regarding unstarted business actually represent two sides of the same coin. While a person has expectations of the "perfect relation," "ideal family," "maximum success," or a "magnificent social life," on one hand, he/she experiences anxieties related with "unrequited love," a "fragmented family," "failure at work," or "social rejection." Such anxieties lead to panic and fear regarding the yet unstarted or unrealized business. The person at this point can neither move toward meeting his/her needs by mobilizing nor give up these needs. This leads to the experience of perpetual restlessness. For example, Steven, who graduated from university two years previously, had been job hunting since then. His goal was to find the best job, with the best pay, in the shortest possible time, and with the greatest ease. However, the jobs he managed to find somehow could not satisfy him in terms of wages, work conditions, hours, or terms, and he did not accept any of them. Hence, for two years, he took no steps toward satisfying either his economic needs or those for success and status. On the other hand, the failure to satisfy these needs made him feel inadequate and good for nothing. Later, Steven found a job that satisfied him in another city, but as he was not sure whether or not he would be content to live in a different city, he again did not accept the job. Meanwhile, as the two-year unemployment started to work against him in his new job applications, his hope of ever finding a good job started to diminish. In the end, Steven applied for therapy as he became unable to leave his home due to feelings of hopelessness, apathy, and insecurity. At the root of his not being able to meet his needs lies his excessive wish to control the future and his catastrophic expectations. Instead of planning how to cope with difficulties, Steven tries not to face them and believes that he would not be able to cope with them.

e. Failure to Use Environmental Alternatives

When new life situations and/or needs emerge, a person first of all has to change his/her former familiar and rigid modes of behavior and to expand his/her behavior repertoire. A wish to continue with old behaviors on one hand and a desire for change and development on the other hand start to stress the person. In order to cope with these hardships and to satisfy his/her needs, it might be necessary for the person to get some support from the environment. For this, the person might have to reevaluate and develop his/her environmental alternatives. Hence, a person in such a situation is at a point where he/she has to investigate and figure out from whom, when, and how he/she can ask for help (Joyce and Sills 2003, 84). Virginia was a person who was generally aware of her need for success, love, to be loved, to participate socially, to stay in good health, and be fit and was successful in prioritizing them according to the situation and time. However, after a while, Virginia's husband had to go out of town frequently and for long periods due to the demands of his work. Their son was greatly affected by this setup and, as he was also entering adolescence, became very tense and rebellious and startedto fail at school. To remedy the situation, Virginia started to dedicate all her time outside of her job to her son and, in time, started losing touch with her friends, her social life, and even her parents. Since she did not have much contact with others, she was not aware that all parents with children of that age live through similar problems and she could not share her feelings and problems about her situation with anybody else. From time to time, she debated getting help from an expert but, believing that as a good and smart mother, she had to solve all her problems herself, did not seek help. On the other hand, she was not considering sharing her feelings with her husband either because she did not want to upset him as he was at home only for short periods. Eventually, all these experiences put her out of sorts, and her relationship with her husband also started to become stressful. She refused her parents' suggestion of leaving the son with them and going to be with her husband for a while, believing that she could not be a good mother if she left her son. Her brother, who was a teacher himself, offered to help with her son's schoolwork but she refused and took on the task of tutoring him by herself. However, this teacher-student relationship further eroded their mother-son relationship. As can be seen from this example, her husband's long-term business trips and her son's entering adolescence has led to problems Virginia could not cope with by herself, but in order to solve them, Virginia instead of using the resources from her environment (such as husband, parents, brother, experts, friends) tried to cope with everything by herself. This ultimately has caused Virginia to feel helpless and unhappy and eventually anxious and pessimistic. In the end, Virginia who could not be of any help to herself, never mind her son, and who found herself in an impasse came for therapy. Virginia's belief that she had to solve everything herself prevented her using environmental alternatives and satisfying her need to cope with her son's problems.

f. Failure to Take Responsibility for One's Needs

One of the factors in the failure to meet needs is the inability of the person to take responsibility for his/her needs. A healthy person is aware of his/her needs, accepts them, and mobilizes to satisfy them (Korb et al. 1989, 51). However, some people instead of making an effort to meet their needs, expect others to do it for them and, when this does not happen, could even accuse them of not responding to their needs. For example, such expressions as "I never take the first step, I always expect others to approach me," "If somebody hurts my feelings, I don't speak to him/her again," "I hate doing things by myself" are indicators of the fact that the person is not making any effort in terms of his/her needs. Likewise, people who declare, "If he/she loves me, then he/she should know what I want without me telling him/her and do it," are those who, instead of meeting their own needs, try to hold others responsible for them. In such cases, by avoiding satisfying his or her own needs, the person renders him/herself a "victim," "helpless," and "weak," but, instead of changing this status and taking on the responsibility for meeting his/her needs, wastes time by accusing the people around him/her.

In summary, in the Gestalt approach, needs and their satisfaction is a crucial subject in terms of both theory and practice. One of the ultimate goals of therapy is to help the client to be aware of his/her needs without judging, to prioritize those needs, to be able to focus on them by identifying with his/her needs, to take on his/her responsibilities in meeting these needs, to be able to use environmental conditions, and eventually to fully satisfy those needs (Perls 1973, 18). The themes and methods to be practiced during therapy in order to help the clients to satisfy their needs are discussed in detail in sections on contact, contact styles, unfinished business, polarities, and resistance.

6

UNFINISHED BUSINESS

One of the most important contributions of the Gestalt approach to the field of psychotherapy is the concept of "unfinished business." This concept is based on two interrelated propositions of the field theory. According to the first of these propositions, humans do not perceive different objects independently from each other; on the contrary, they perceive them by organizing them into a meaningful whole. If you look at the examples below, you will notice that the first is perceived as a triangle and the second one as rectangle rather than separate dots.

● ● ●

● ● ● ●

Now look at the other figures. You will notice that you do not perceive them as various splotches.

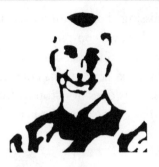

A man

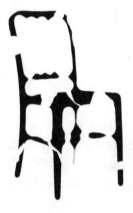

A chair

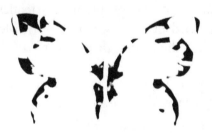

A butterfly

You will see a man in the first figure and a chair in the second. To recognize anything in the third figure is a little more difficult. However, when carefully looked at, you will see that it is a butterfly.

According to the second proposition of the field theory, people tend to complete what is missing. For example, when we see an incomplete circle, such as the one below, we complete it in our minds and perceive it as a circle. What can you see in the second picture? A cat, isn't it? Maybe you did not notice at first glance, but this cute little cat is missing its tail and an ear. Nevertheless, this does not stop us from perceiving it as a cat because we complete what is missing in our minds.

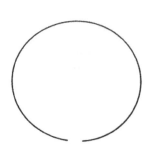 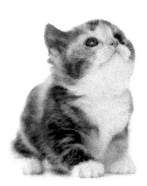

Zeigarnik (1927), starting from these propositions put forth by the Gestalt psychologists depending on the perception studies they carried out in the 1920s, has shown with his experimental studies that people remember unfinished business better than the finished ones. His experiments greatly contributed to the development of unfinished business concept of the Gestalt approach and were included in Gestalt books as the "Zeigarnik effect." Ovsiankina (1928) took his experimental studies further and stated that people have a tendency to go back to complete the unfinished business spontaneously. Moving on from the results of these studies, the Gestalt therapy approach has concluded that

a. People have a tendency to finish their formerly unfinished business (their needs, contacts, or feelings),

b. They do not forget them until they are finished,

c. They search for a variety of ways to finish them.

In the Gestalt approach, the concept of unfinished business is related to the failure of a person to meet his/her needs in a satisfactory manner. When a person cannot meet these needs satisfactorily, the Gestalt cannot be completed and remains half done. The incomplete Gestalt can emerge in two ways. The first is that the Gestalt remains open to be completed, and the second is the closing of the Gestalt without completion, that is, fixation of the Gestalt. A discussion of these two cases in which the Gestalt is not completed satisfactorily is given in the following section.

The Meaning of Unfinished Business

As mentioned before, people are more at ease, peaceful, and happy the easier, faster, and more satisfactorily they meet their needs. However, there is no doubt that it is not always possible for a person to meet all his/her needs either in a short time or completely satisfactorily. In such situations, we are left with a lot of unmet needs and with much unfinished business. People generally try to complete those tasks they think are more important or more pleasant as soon as possible and postpone the others. For example, in order to meet your girlfriend or boyfriend, you may easily postpone your homeworks that should be done or going somewhere that you should but do not really want to. In another instance, you might delay going to the dentist for your routine checkup as long as you experience no pain, and perhaps even when you do. Some people act in exactly the opposite way and give priority to completing those tasks they see as mandatory or meet the needs of others; however, in that case, they fail to meet their personal needs. In the end, the unfinished business, whether it is an unpaid bill, a call not made, a sweater not bought or homework not done, depending on the importance and the urgency of the need in question, occupies the mind of the person and bothers him/her. As the amount of unfinished business increases, the person not only feels tense but also starts feeling inadequate, tired, and burned out.

No matter how tiring and energy consuming the failure to complete the daily tasks may be, actually the unfinished business that causes problems is the ones related to the conflicts experienced with those people who are important for us. Such conflicts may lead us to feel pain, sorrow, sadness, hurt, anger, resentment, hate, shame, or guilt. In such cases, the need to be met should be the expression of these feelings, thereby sharing them and then resolving the conflict. Some people, particularly at the end of conflicts they experience with those close to them, sulk and may continue this silence for days, even weeks. By sulking, they obstruct the expression of their feelings and thoughts as well as those of the other party and cause some unfinished business among them to remain. Sulking has a vastly different meaning to terminating a relationship. In a terminated relationship, the parties no longer have any expectations from each other. In contrast, sulking indicates that the person has some expectations from the other side and that the fulfillment of these expectations is deferred. Hence, sulking is one of the best examples that can be given to unfinished business. The person who sulks cannot release his/her energy because he/she is unable to express the unfinished feelings, and this unreleased energy builds up and leads to outbursts of anger or physical disturbances with psychological roots. Because of this, in conflict situations, instead of sulking, expressing the feelings in an appropriate way should be the way forward. Some people, without resolving the conflict, act as if nothing has happened. They decide to give themselves another chance or to "turn over a new leaf." However, to make such a decision when the previous feelings and thoughts have not been shared appropriately, when those to be forgiven have not been discussed, and when those to be accepted are still awaiting acceptance actually means that a lot of unfinished business remains in this relationship. This failure to finish the unfinished business leads to the reemergence of former conflicts at the earliest opportunity. In some cases, unfinished business may stem from an event experienced or witnessed in the past such as abuse, rape, violence, terrorism, or war, from being exposed to an earthquake, flood, or fire, or from having an accident, illness, or operation. Furthermore, life experiences that cause a person to feel guilt or shame in particular can also remain as unfinished. For example, if life experiences such as being excluded by a group or an important person or being seen while masturbating or hearing unpleasant remarks about one's body can still cause very intense feelings when remembered despite the passing of years, then this means they are unfinished.

The unfinished business mentioned here concerns those memories that can be recalled that means they are related not to a very distant past. Therefore, they can be completed when the person is ready to confront his/her feelings. However, in particular, those childhood experiences that cause negative feelings such as pain, sadness, hurt, fear, revenge, hate, guilt, or shame are not remembered and lead to the formation of fixed Gestalts.

Fixed Gestalt

A young child, inadequately equipped, cannot deal in a healthy manner with the intense feelings caused by traumatic and difficult life experiences faced in his/her childhood and, in order to get rid of these negative emotions, gives up attempting to satisfy his/her needs. In other words, as the child cannot satisfactorily complete the Gestalt he/she has created to meet his/her needs because of intense negative feelings, he/she closes it "prematurely" and "inappropriately." In the Gestalt approach, this is known as fixation of the Gestalt.

Fixation of a Gestalt leads to the obstruction of natural reactions and the replacement of these reactions by others (Sills et al. 1998, 73). For example, every time Bob felt sad and cried, his parents instead of approaching him with indulgence, trying to understand the causes of his sadness and then calming him down, reacted angrily, commenting, "Big boys don't cry." On the other hand, Bob's bold and aggressive behaviors were praised, particularly by his father, with appreciative comments such as "Look at my courageous boy," or "Men should be bold and strong like this." As such reactions became repetitive, Bob first started not to cry when he was feeling sad, then not to articulate his sadness, then not to notice it, and finally to express it as anger. Hence, for Bob, the pattern of getting angry instead of feeling sad became a fixed Gestalt. Gaby, on the other hand, whenever she was naughty was scolded and sent to her room by her parents with comments such as "Come back when you have learnt how to behave." Alone in her room, feeling lonely and guilty, Gaby did not know what to do, and to calm herself, she would tidy her drawers or arrange her toys in a strict order. After being sent to her room like this many times, Gaby developed a fixed Gestalt, and at first, every time she felt lonely and guilty and later, without even being aware of the feelings she was experiencing, she started to tidy the drawers in her room even when they were in good order and to continuously check whether or not the furniture and objects were in their assigned places. Gaby eventually became a very irritable mother who could not tolerate the slightest untidiness in the house and who mistreated her husband and children because of their being messy. When Catherine needed love and attention from her mother, her mother would often say, "I am very busy, I can't deal with you now," "Don't bother me, I am in a bad mood," or just "Go away and leave me alone." As her need to be loved and cared for remained unsatisfied, Catherine tried to alleviate the hurt and sadness she felt by holding her breath and straining her chest muscles. Faced with such remarks again and again, Catherine eventually fixated her "hunchback" posture, spoke in a very low voice, and became an introvert. As these three examples demonstrate, Bob with his temper, Gaby with her over fastidiousness, and Catherine with her poor posture have been trying to protect themselves from feeling bad and getting hurt. As their needs to be loved and cared for remained unmet for long periods, in the course of time, they could not even remember what their original needs were. Those children whose needs were ignored by their families eventually learnt to ignore their own emotional needs.

Fixed Gestalts or, in other words, the ways the child developed in order to avoid hurt and mistreatment, determine his/her way of existence in later years, that is, his/her physical, emotional, behavioral, and cognitive processes (Clarkson and Mackewn 1993, 69). Hence, the person whose unfinished needs are fixed, even if his/her present environment is greatly different than the one in his/her childhood, continues to react just like he/she did as a child and tries to satisfy the unmet needs of childhood in the present. Actually, having a person try to meet these needs, even if unconsciously, and showing an effort to satisfy the unmet needs of the past now is a very healthy attitude. In this way, the person is trying to solve the problems of the past. However, as the Gestalt is fixed, the person cannot meet those needs both because he/she is still not fully aware of them and is also still using the old and dysfunctional ways to satisfy them. For example, in his interpersonal relations, Bob, by reacting with anger instead of telling those around him what hurts him, eliminates the possibility of being understood and treated with consideration. Gaby, instead of playing with her children and having a pleasant time with her husband, by constantly putting her home in order and by even being angry with her family's untidiness, loses the chance of their being closer and more affectionate to her. Catherine, instead of being with people and establishing contact, by giving an impression of being closed to communication with her "hunchback" posture and very low voice and by not meeting other people very often anyway, cannot get the love and attention she craves. For all these reasons, Bob, Gaby, and Catherine can't meet their needs or complete their Gestalts. In other words, because of the fixed Gestalt, the person knows neither which needs to satisfy nor how. Due to the fixed Gestalt, the person's physical, emotional, behavioral, and cognitive reactions are so far away from his/her original needs that it becomes very difficult to see the connection between these reactions and the needs. The person is so used to this fixed Gestalt that he/she is really not aware of what he/she is doing, how he/she is doing it, or for what purpose. Thus, the symptoms that occur are generally covert and seem independent of the unfinished business.

The Consequences of Unfinished Business

As the unfinished business forces the person to be finished, it does not disappear into the background like finished business or completed Gestalts. On the contrary, it remains constantly in the background and continuously waits for an opportunity to become a figure. This causes a constant shift between the figure and the ground and thus prevents the person from focusing on the present moment and new experiences. Clarkson (1991, 7) explains this with a story whose author is anonymous. When a famous composer (Mozart or Beethoven, according to the version) went to bed one night to sleep, he heard that his downstairs neighbor was playing a concerto on the piano. The neighbor, despite performing beautifully, somehow could never manage to complete the final chords and kept returning to the beginning. Although the composer was very tired, he could not sleep while this was going on. In the end, he got out of bed, played the closing bars himself, and having finished the incomplete auditory gestalt, he was able to sleep. Many of us experience similar incidents and situations. For example, when we are waiting for important news or if we are bothered about something, we cannot listen to the people around us attentively, no matter how interesting their conversation is. Similarly, we may sometimes reflect negative feelings that are due to another similar but previous situation or person onto those who are around us. One of the best examples of this is those people who, no matter who they are angry with, take out their anger on those they encounter in traffic. Polster and Polster (1974, 37) have pointed out that unfinished business can cause symptoms such as inability to concentrate, forgetfulness, labile mind, and in the severest cases, manic psychosis. Clarkson and Mackewn (1993, 69), on the other hand, claimed that unfinished business plays a crucial role in the development of neurotic symptoms and neurotic character.

Unfinished business can make the person answer questions such as "What happened?" "What did he say?" "What did I say?" "What did I do?" or "How did I do that?" over and over again, leading to mental repetitions. For example, some students, after taking an important examination, continuously go over their answers until the results are announced. When performed frequently and intensely, these mental repetitions might lead to obsessions. Similarly, unfinished business might lead to compulsions, that is, repetitive acts such as cleaning, washing, and checking things. In obsessions and compulsions, the figure and ground do not change places, and unfinished business becomes a steady figure but never can be completed (Polster and Polster 1974, 36). Mental repetitions when done frequently and intensely can also cause physical tensions. Korb et al. (1989, 64) have pointed out that symptoms such as ulcers, stress headaches, neck and back pains, arthritis, and asthma can also be related to unfinished business. The effects of unfinished business can be seen most obviously in post-traumatic stress disorder. The person who was traumatized, in order to be able to tolerate it, shows a tendency toward not remembering it and suppressing his/her feelings about it. Hence, the experienced trauma remains as unfinished business and starts to affect negatively the current life of the person.

Sometimes the unfinished business can be related to a specific subject such as sexuality, beauty, or success. In such cases, the person determines his/her whole life according to this unfinished business and is constantly involved with it. When the person directs all his/her energy to the unfinished subject, then there remains no energy for new and different ones.

How to Work with Unfinished Business in Therapy

While working with unfinished business in therapy, the aim is

1. To have the client become aware of his/her unfinished business,
2. To have the client reach underlying needs by reexperiencing his/her memories related to the unfinished business,

3. To have the client express his/her related feelings,

4. To have the client accomplish alternative ways and skills to satisfy these needs in his/her current life.

When the client completes his/her unfinished business in a healthy way, then it will be possible to direct his/her blocked energy to "now" and "new" experiences.

Some clients have so much unfinished business that they don't know which complaint they should start with. In that case, the therapist should start working with the complaints that are most important for the client and investigate to see if there is a connection with the complaints and the unfinished business of the client. Here the starting point should be the clients' relationships with their kin and people who have had a significant place in their life. Later, the memories that seem most important to the client should be determined and they should be relived as if they were being experienced at that moment. During this act of recall, the client should be helped to become aware of his/her feelings, thoughts, and posture. The purpose of this work is to determine how the unfinished business originally appeared, or in other words, to find out the history of the unfinished business. For example, one of the clearest memories Judith could recollect was the scene where her father was beating her older brother, her mother was crying in a corner, and she was hiding under the table and watching them. Such scenes were frequently repeated during Judith's childhood. While Judith was reliving this scene during therapy, the upper part of her body was leaning forward, her shoulders were raised, and there were tears in her eyes. During the work, she became aware that she used to feel very scared and helpless in this scene.

Once the history of the unfinished business is determined, then work is carried out on the physical, emotional, behavioral, and cognitive effects of these memories on the current existence of the client. Judith, who is mentioned above, was a very successful high-ranking administrator. During her school years, she was also a very successful and well-adjusted child; she never caused any trouble for her family, and she was proud of this. When she applied for therapy, she had been married for ten years and she was the mother of two children. She had no problems in her relations with her friends and children but had serious problems in her marriage and was suffering from back pains and headaches. Recently, she had been feeling lonely and tired, could not sleep because of her pains, and was having difficulty in concentrating. Her husband had started to keep away from home and acted in a hostile manner. Judith did not talk about her problems with anybody and was exerting extra effort so that her parents and children would not notice her difficulties.

Underneath unfinished business, "introjected" messages play a significant role. Consequently during therapy, work should also be carried out to define these introjections. How this can be done is explained in detail in the section on "introjections." During therapy, it became apparent that the introjected message that most affected Judith's current behavior was "Stand on your own feet and do not cause any trouble." While Judith was watching the scenes between her father and brother and the helplessness of her mother, she realized that nobody was in a state where they could pay her any attention, so she "decided" that she should not cause any further problems and tried to satisfy the love and attention she needed by not causing any trouble and even by trying to patch things up among them. In this way, even though she satisfied her need for success and appreciation, she never met her need to "act and to be liked as she is".

In the Gestalt approach, one of the techniques that can be used for the completion of unfinished business is empty or two-chair exercises. The chair experiments enable the client to engage in a monologue or dialogue with the person or persons who have caused him/her to experience negative feelings either in his/her daily life, near past or childhood, and to express these feelings and thoughts to them. To put this process into motion, the client is first asked to choose a person who caused him/her negative feelings, to imagine that person as sitting in the empty chair, and then to express his/her feelings and thoughts about that person. In some cases, two-chair experiments are more useful. In these experiments once the client talks about his/her feelings and thoughts to the person sitting in the empty chair, then he/she moves to that chair and answers her previous comments in the role of that person. Empty and two-chair experiments provide an opportunity for clients to express themselves much better, as well as giving them a chance to unburden all their feelings. During these exercises, pillows can also be used. A pillow might be put in the empty chair resembling the person to whom the client is expressing his/her feelings. In this way the client can express his/her anger to the other person by hitting the pillow or his/her positive feelings by hugging it.

While working with Judith during therapy, it became apparent that she had unfinished business not only with her parents but also with her older brother. In one session, Judith talked about how, despite he is only two years older than she, they could never be close, how there were periods of extreme tension between them due to her brother's aggressive behavior and how she felt regret after his sudden death because of this lack of closeness. At this point, Judith was asked to imagine that she was at her brother's grave and to have a dialogue with him. A part of the two-chair experiment related to the unfinished business between Judith and her older brother is given below.

Therapist:	*What would you like to say to your brother?*
Judith:	*I don't know what to say to you because I never really knew you. You got married very young and left home. But you were always very bad tempered. No matter what I did, I could never please you. But I always wanted you to be a good brother to me. I would like to tell you my troubles. I wanted you to guide me, protect me and support me. I don't know what I have done to deserve your mistreatment* (tears started to fall)
Judith (as her brother):	I don't know. You made me angry. Always talking like miss-know-it-all. You never gave any grief to our parents and that drove me crazy. I was the one getting the beatings because of my low grades. You were a good student. You were quiet. You made me feel bad about myself. We could never have anything in common.

Judith:	(crying) *You always had problems, always bad tempered. You gave my mother so much grief; you made her cry many times. You only cared about yourself. You were irresponsible most of the time. You were just shouting. I couldn't connect with you. I didn't know what to say or how to say it.*
Judith (as her brother):	*Yes, because everything made me angry.* My father was always angry with me. He never trusted me, even when I was trying to do something good. And my mother was always crying out of the blue. You were always studying or busy with something, never on my side. (After a period of silence)
Therapist:	*What are you feeling right now?*
Judith:	(crying and kneeling on the floor) *I am so sorry. I wish we could have found a way to talk. I am really sorry about this. I never realized things were like this. Rest in peace. I hope you have calmed down there and your anger has gone.*
Therapist:	*What is your brother saying?*
Judith (as her brother):	*I don't know what to say, but I was not* happy. Particularly in the last year. But I always followed you from a distance. I wanted you to be well, and I was proud of you, even though I did not show it.
Judith:	*I didn't really know you well, but a lot of people said such wonderful things about you at your funeral. Then I was also proud of you. I wish I also had something to say* (sobbing). *Farewell brother. I can't say I will miss you, but I wish we had been closer. I wish we were really a brother and a sister.*

In such two-chair experiments, the purpose is to have the person express his/her feelings, thoughts, and needs. They are not practice sessions for a real life conversation. Furthermore, in two-chair work, knowing what the person occupying the opposite chair might say in reality has no importance. What is important is what the person initiating the dialogue guesses about what the other person might say. As can be seen from the above example, empty-chair or two-chair techniques are very useful in completion of the unfinished business of the clients with people who have died, who live far away, or those whom they do not want to face. In some cases, in order to complete unfinished business, the client might need to have a dialogue with the other person in his/her daily life. If the client is avoiding such an encounter, then the reasons for this should be explored. During the therapy, if necessary, different modes of conversation could also be acted out through the two-chair technique.

No experience that has led to intense negative feelings can be wholly completed, that is, it cannot become unlived. However, with the work carried out in therapy, clients can come to a level that does not hurt as much as before, and the negative effects on the person's current life can be alleviated. In order to achieve this, the person first has to accept what happened in the past as it is, forgive those involved, and then to integrate with these experiences. When integration is achieved, then the person starts to be able to focus on the now and to meet his/her needs in different ways than those used in the past. For example Judith, after the two-chair work she carried out with her brother, started to meet with her brother's son, from whom she had been estranged, just as she had been from her brother. This, no doubt, did not change her relation with her brother, but to see her nephew and to get to know him a little better made it easier for her to forgive her brother as well as herself.

In conclusion, the purpose of work related with unfinished business during therapy is, by eliminating the negative effects of the past, to help the client to live the present fully and satisfactorily. The person who has completed his/her unfinished business has learned to establish better contact with both other people and him/herself, to participate in life more energetically and more actively, and most important of all, to be aware of his/her needs, to articulate them properly, and to find the ways of satisfying them. However, completion of unfinished business is a tough process because all the negative feelings such as anger, guilt, shame, or sorrow, which were avoided in the past, are relived and experienced during therapy. Hence, resistance can occur during work on unfinished business, and this is normal. Because of this, during the completion of unfinished business during therapy, in addition to styles of contact, it might be necessary to work on the client's resistances, impasses and polarities. Theoretical and practical information on such work will be given in the following sections.

7

CONTACT

One of the points that distinguish the Gestalt approach from other therapy approaches is its emphasis on the concept of contact. The concept of contact carries serious significance for the Gestalt approach because of the role it plays in the emergence of psychological problems and in ensuring growth and change. Contact is experienced on the contact boundary between the organism and the environment. In this regard, it is possible to say that the real focal points of the Gestalt therapy approach are the contact of the client with him/herself, with his/her physical and social environment, and with the therapist. In order to establish effective contact, all the contact paths must be open and the contact boundary must be flexible and permeable. The person fulfils his/her needs by establishing contact with the environment and withdrawing afterward in a rhythmic way. The rhythm is determined by the contact styles. The individual and the environment are equally responsible for disruption in the rhythm of contact and withdrawal. Rhythm disruption occurs when the needs of the individual and the society differ from each other and when the individual cannot decide whether his/her own needs or those of society are more important. The concept of contact as viewed by the Gestalt approach is explained in detail in the sections below.

Contact Is Experienced on the Contact Boundary between the Organism and Its Environment

According to the Gestalt approach, the person and the environment should be taken as a whole, because without establishing contact with the environment, one cannot satisfy his/her needs and thus cannot survive. If people were to be in state of solitude, they would have had little chance to survive physically. In this state of loneliness, survival in the psychological and emotional sense would have been even less likely. Just as the individual is in need of air, food, and drink on a physiological level, he/she is in need of other individuals on a psychological level. Perls (1973, 25) noted that for humankind, the sense of identification is the primary psychological survival impulse.

Hence, it is not possible to keep the person and the environment separate from each other and deal with them individually. Perls (1973, 17) explains this with the following example: The sentence "I see a tree" can be divided into subject, object, and verb. However, this experience of seeing a tree cannot be divided into parts because, in order to see the tree, both the tree and the person are needed. As other therapeutic approaches try to separate the person and the environment from one another, they are stuck on the unresolved question of whether the individual is ruled by internal or external forces. According to Perls (1973, 16) this kind of question derives from the need to give a causal explanation. However, just for the sake of giving causal explanations, not paying attention to the relations between the organism and the environment leads to numerous problems. Examining solely the individual's organismic structure is the subject of anatomy and physiology. Examining solely the environment is the subject of physical, social, and geographical sciences. By evaluating the organism and the environment separately and independently, these sciences fall into an illusion "as if an eye has the power to affect the object it sees or as if an object has the power to affect the eyes that stare at it." According to the Gestalt approach, by addressing the person in his/her environment, psychology must focus on the boundary where the contact between the person and the environment is established, because all thoughts, behaviors, actions, and emotions are determined by this contact (Perls 1973, 17).

Thus, the Gestalt approach sees the human being as a function of the organism and its environment and believes that thoughts, behaviors, actions, and emotions are all determined by the contact between the two. Hence, in accordance with this perspective, it regards the person both as an individual and as a social being. Every human being has his/her own unique needs and has to meet these needs from the physical and social environment. In order to do this, the individual has two innate features. The first one is being able to sense which outside objects will satisfy their needs (Perls 1973, 17). For example, when a baby is hungry, it will directly go to its mother's breast without paying any attention to the shapes, smells, sounds, and colors around. The second feature is to have a sense of physical, psychological, and social balance, or in other words, to have a tendency to form a balance between one's own needs and physical and social demands. For instance, when the baby is unable to reach to its mother's breast, it will then turn toward the baby bottle in order to satisfy its hunger. In other words, an individual can satisfy his/her needs according to the conditions offered by the environment. Experience is a function of the contact boundary between the organism and the environment. The contact boundary is the place where the person experiences "me" in relation to "not me." A person's self-boundary is determined by previous and new experiences (Polster and Polster 1974, 108). All psychological phenomena occur on this contact boundary. Put it another way, the contact boundary is the place where the individual differentiates from and meets other individuals (Clarkson and Mackewn 1993, 56). The choices made at the boundary determine lifestyle, nature of the chosen community, work experience, home, family, and/or love relations (Korb et al. 1989, 33). Thus, the contact boundary belongs to both the organism and the environment. Therefore, the contact boundary is not static; instead it has a dynamic structure and changes from moment to moment according to the changes in the person, environment, and the person-environment interaction.

Growth and Change Can Only Be Achieved through Contact

The reason for the concept of contact having particular importance in the Gestalt therapy approach is the belief that the only way an individual can grow and change is through contact (Clarkson and Mackewn 1993, 55). Contact, as has been seen, is the meeting of the person with other people and the environment (Perls 1951/1996, 30–72). In brief, every kind of relationship between the person and the environment, such as eating, running, feeling, screaming, laughing, hugging, fighting, loving, and the like, is a form of contact. As can be understood from this definition, more than one person, object, or condition is necessary for contact to take place. Thus, contact can only occur between two or more different things. Thence, contact is the relationship between "me" and "not me" or the differentiation of "I" and "you." Contact involves some kind of exchange. During contact, whether metaphoric or real, something is "received" from outside and is "given" out. This receiving and giving emerges from the attraction or repulsion between two clearly delineated and discriminated things (Korb et al. 1989, 33). For example, when you meet someone, greeting him/her, chatting, grimacing, or avoiding looking at him/her are forms of contact. Contact extends into interaction with inanimate as well as animate objects (Polster and Polster 1974, 102). Staring at a tree, watching the sunset, hearing the sounds of birds, and listening to the silence of a cave are all in themselves forms of contact. An individual can make contact with him/herself as well (Korb et al. 1989, 33). Recalling memories or imagining the future can be given as examples of establishing contact with oneself.

Just as we may not be aware of gravity when we walk, we may not always be aware of the contacts we make. We may be aware of what we say, what we see, or what we hear when talking with someone, but we may not be aware of the actual contact we are experiencing. These kinds of "unaware" contacts do not lead to growth or change. For growth and change to occur, the contact must be alive and dynamic; that is to say, the person has to be active and creative during contact. As a result of such contact, some aspects of the personality and the features of the environment are integrated and this leads to a new, enlarged and different sense of self (Clarkson and Mackewn 1993, 55).

According to Perls et al. (1951/1996, 230), contact leads to the new behavior through the acceptance of the assimilable novelty and the rejection of the inassimilable novelty. In other words, whether or not it is assimilable, an individual that makes contact with the environment inevitably changes, because contact is implicitly incompatible with remaining the same. According to Polster and Polster (1974, 101), through contact, one does not have to try to change; change simply occurs. Contact is the cornerstone of change and provides the vital energy for enabling such change. However, what kind of change is going to occur cannot be known or predicted beforehand. Change can also be harmful and destructive for the individual (Korb et al. 1989, 33).

In Order to Achieve Good Contact, the Pathways of Contact Have to Be Open

Individuals establish the contact with the environment primarily through their sensory organs, namely, eyes, ears, nose, mouth, and skin. These sensory organs determine the contact boundary and give information that enables the person to function in a healthy way (Korb et al. 1989, 39). Two other ways of contact are talking and movement. Whether or not the contact will lead to change and growth is determined by whether or not these pathways of contact are used and, if so, how they are used. The contact is made using one or more of the pathways depending on the circumstances. Now each of these pathways will be investigated.

Seeing

One of the routes to establish contact is seeing. Individuals without visual impairment can see everything around them if their eyes are open and if there is enough light in the environment. However, this alone is insufficient for contact. In order to establish contact, the person has to be willing to see, aware of what he/she sees, and able to give meaning to it. In other words, for contact, it is not enough to look: to really see is necessary. Although in our daily lives we see dozens of objects, people, sights, and so on, we do not establish contact with most of them. For example, we don't establish eye contact with other people sometimes because we don't give importance to them, sometimes intentionally and sometimes otherwise. Another way of obstructing contact is staring at someone for a long time. Just as our hands and feet get numb and insentient if we remain in the same position for too long, staring at someone for a long time also causes numbness or, in other words, prevents us from being aware of what we are seeing.

Hearing

Another way of establishing contact is hearing. Individuals without hearing impairment can hear the sounds or silence around them. Just as in seeing, hearing is not enough on its own to establish contact. In order to establish contact, the person has to be willing to hear, make sense of what he/she hears, and react accordingly. Because some people are very sensitive to criticism, they have a strong tendency to hear only the negative expressions and ignore the positive ones. Some people only hear what they want to hear. Some people who are afraid of quarrels cannot bear loud noises; some people can't sleep in the presence of even the lowest level of noise. A person's tone of voice is very important in establishing contact with others because the voice plays an important role in expressing emotions. For instance, in Japanese Kabuki theatre, words are not used; instead of words various sounds are used to express the meaning of the play. Some people talk in a mechanical way with no ups and downs in the tone of their voice. Furthermore, speaking either in a very high or low tone or talking breathlessly or intermittently can obstruct contact. However, the most frequent problem related to hearing is misunderstanding of what is being heard.

Talking

Talking is very closely connected with listening in terms of contact. The properties of the language being used are also important in establishing contact. For example, some people use enriched and colorful language. Some people have poor vocabulary to express their feelings. Some people get lost in details and thus have difficulty in focusing on the subject matter. Some people, by constantly repeating the same sentences, others by talking in a generalized or abstract way, bore the listener. Some use jargon too often and confuse the listener. Some people do not use subjects in their sentences and make it impossible to understand about whom they are talking. Some people talk without pausing; others cannot find anything to say. All of the abovementioned talking patterns obstruct contact.

Another way in which the contact is obstructed is giving double messages while talking. Some people frequently play the game of "yes, but . . ." For example, phrases like "yes, you look beautiful, but your lipstick is too red," "very well cooked, but it's too salty," or "yes, the dress fits you well, but the back of it seems a little odd" make it difficult for the listener to choose which part of the sentence to believe. In other words, the person cannot decide whether she should think that she does not look beautiful because she put on lipstick that is too red or to focus on the first part of the sentence and believe she looks beautiful. Instead of using direct sentences, some people communicate through questions. For example, they ask, "Do you really like him?" in such a tone that it is understood that what they are trying achieve is not to get a straight answer but to obscure their true meaning, which is along the lines of, "I don't really like him and you shouldn't either. If you do, I'll be upset." Or when they ask, "Are you coming?" they really mean "I hope you are not coming." Some people prefer to use "you" instead of "I." For example, when people say, "You feel sad in situations like these" or "These kinds of talks annoy people," they actually mean that "I feel sad in situations like these" or "These kinds of talks annoy me." In this way, they do not take responsibility for their own feelings but generalize their own feelings to others.

Laughing is also another way of establishing contact. Not to laugh at all, to laugh in an exaggerated manner, to laugh at everything, to laugh silently or with a closed mouth, to laugh with a very high-pitched tone or to force oneself to laugh may disrupt the establishment of contact.

Touching

In everyday language, "touch" is the first word that comes to mind associated with the word "contact." Handshaking, hugging, caressing, kissing, pushing, and hitting are among the most frequently used physical forms of touching. Even though touching is one of our five senses, actually it is the center of them all (Polster and Polster 1974, 129). For example, seeing is being touched by light waves whereas hearing is being touched by sound waves. Smelling and tasting are being touched by chemicals, either gaseous or in solution. By listening to each other, looking at each other, or talking with each other, we actually "touch" one another. Phrases we use such as "The way he looked at me touched me," "What he said really touched me," and "We have remained in touch with her for years" emphasize the importance of various forms of touch in establishing contact.

As touching covers all other ways of contact and as there is a little or no distance during touching, contact by touching is more effective. That is why there are many rules and prohibitions regarding touching. For example, "Don't touch valuable objects," "Don't touch your genitals," "Don't touch other people," and "Don't touch dirty things" are a few of the most common prohibitions. All societies have their own rules regarding with whom one can shake hands, with whom one can walk hand in hand or arm in arm, whom one can kiss, hug, hit, or punch.

The style of handshake is also important in terms of contact. Some establish contact with a firm handshake, whilst others shake with the tips of their fingers. Some people avoid kissing even those who are close to them. Whilst some people avoid kissing women, others avoid kissing men. Moreover, some people tend to touch very often as they talk, while others put a distance and don't want to touch at all. All of these behavior patterns affect contact.

Smelling

Although it may not have as apparent an impact as other forms of contact, smelling is still considered to have importance as a way of contact. While some people are very sensitive to scents, others are only affected by foul smells. Perfumes, without a doubt, emphasize the importance of smelling in our daily life. The smell of fresh coffee in a cold day, the smell of food when we are hungry, or the smell of the flowers we share with loved ones can also be important in terms of establishing contact with our environment.

Tasting

Tasting is one of the ways we use to achieve contact, especially with food and beverages. Some people eat while watching TV or while walking; some swallow without chewing, and some eat very slowly and chew extensively. Some of us like to eat sweets; some of us like savory, and others like spicy food. Whilst some people feel every taste in their mouth, it is difficult for some people to be aware of different tastes.

Moving

Using the body is another way to establish contact. Some people use their body in a flexible and spontaneous way; whereas others prefer to keep it under control and have a more tense and stiff body. Some people walk very upright, some walk unsteadily, some walk as if leaping, some with their shoulders upfront, and some walk with their belly proudly in front. Some sit by closing their legs, some keep them wide open, and others squat down. All these walking and sitting patterns affect our contact with others in a different way.

For Good Contact, the Contact Boundary Must be Flexible and Permeable

Psychologically healthy individuals are in good contact both with themselves and their environment. People who are able to establish contact are aware of the boundary between themselves and their environment and are able to decide with whom, what, and when to establish contact. These individuals are open to contact, and their self-boundaries are flexible and permeable. In other words, the contact boundary is as flexible and permeable as I boundary of an individual allows. The flexibility and permeability of each person's boundaries are different from those of another. Some people can easily make significant changes in their I boundaries and thus "grow" rapidly. These people not only gain self-confidence by achieving their desires through their own efforts but also are able to respond dynamically and effectively in situations that are either totally or partially out of their control.

Successful individuals are those who have flexible I boundaries. Some people are closed to contact; they do not expand their I boundaries and thus cannot grow and change. Individuals with these kinds of rigid, stereotypical behaviors can neither establish nor sustain good contact. People who are constantly worried about the future and try to control everything have thick and rigid I boundaries. These people are very scared of taking risks, trying out new things, and going in different directions. They are so entrapped in their I boundaries that even the thought of expanding these boundaries may cause panic and anxiety. Whenever they encounter a difficulty, they start to feel weak, empty, unsuccessful, and hopeless. For instance, if a person who is separated from his/her partner continuously spends his time getting angry with that person, pitying him/herself or feeling anxious about the future instead of finding a new life, new harmony, or a new lover, etc., this indicates that this person is not expanding but narrowing his/her I boundaries.

I boundary can also be described from different perspectives such as body boundaries, value boundaries, familiarity boundaries, expression boundaries, and exposure boundaries (Polster and Polster 1974, 115). For instance, those who have flexible body boundaries try to be aware of all parts of their bodies, care for their bodily needs, and use their bodies spontaneously and easily. On the other hand, those who have rigid body boundaries can only be aware of sensations that come from certain parts of their bodies and avoid awareness of certain other parts (e.g. erogenous zones) and functions of the body. Value boundaries may also prevent good contact from being established. For instance, those who have value judgments such as, "Being tidy and clean must be more important than anything else," "People should always think about their loved ones first," or "Women are weak," cannot satisfy their needs with ease. Habits also contribute to the rigidity of the contact boundary. Some people are so dependent on their habits that they do not want to change their jobs, friends, relations, or even the newspaper they read despite being unsatisfied with them. They are afraid of experimenting with something new, and in order to find justifications for their habits, they use expressions such as "Is the new one going to be any better?" "You'll miss the old when the new comes," or "You can't teach an old dog new tricks," and in this way, they exhibit how determined they are not to change their habits. Expressive boundaries are another significant factor in terms of contact. Some families forbid their children to express their feelings and needs from very early ages. For example, children who grow up with bans such as "Don't cry," "Don't shout," "Don't make demands," "Don't laugh too much," "Don't run," and even "Don't have fun" learn not only to restrict themselves but also to avoid those who cry, shout, make demands, laugh, run, or have fun. Finally, the exposure boundary is about drawing the attention of others and being noticed by them. People who have strict exposure boundaries are afraid of putting themselves forward, whether in a negative or positive way. As they do not want to be criticized, they might avoid talking; as they do not want to be pitied, they might not tell their worries and concerns, or as they do not want to tempt fate, they might keep their positive experiences to themselves. All these actions prevent them from establishing close relations with other individuals. Lack of flexibility and permeability of boundaries play an important role in the emergence of all sorts of psychological disorders but especially in depression and anxiety.

Contact and Withdrawal Are a Rhythm

When a person is aware of a need through his/her senses, he/she establishes contact with the environment in order to make the necessary regulations and arrangements to fulfill this need. Once the need is satisfied, the person withdraws by ending the contact. For example, one will stop eating when feeling full, one who misses a friend hangs up the phone after talking and relieving his/her longing, a student who successfully passes an exam will not study any longer. Later, when another need emerges, the person once again establishes contact with the environment to satisfy this need and then withdraws. This is called the contact and withdrawal rhythm. In other words, contact and withdrawal allow us to satisfy our needs in a rhythmic pattern. The contact and withdrawal rhythm can be shown as below:

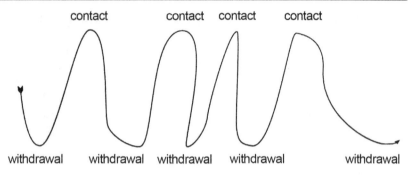

The contact and withdrawal rhythm shown as a wave (Mackewn 1999, 21)

Contact-withdrawal rhythm, which is determined according to the needs and means of satisfying these needs, can be disrupted in two ways. The first is being in the contact or withdrawal phase for a long time. If contact is sustained for too long, it will lose its effectiveness and even become disturbing. For example, if you eat too much, the food will lose its taste and your stomach will be upset; if you spend too much time on the phone with your friends, you will eventually run out of things to say and pay high telephone bills; if you study too much, your brain may become overloaded and you will get confused. On the other hand, if withdrawal lasts too long, that is to say, if you do not eat, meet your friends, or study at all, then you may start feeling physically, psychologically, and socially bad, and this may even result in death.

The questions below can be helpful in determining whether the contact and withdrawal rhythm of the person is healthy or pathological.

With whom and with what does the person establish contact? For how long does the person establish contact?

How does the person establish contact?

From whom and from what does the person withdraw? For how long does the person withdraw?

How does the person withdraw?

Another way in which the rhythm of contact and withdrawal is disrupted is being able to experience fully neither the contact nor the withdrawal phase. For example, being distracted while talking to someone or listening to something, not being able to get away from someone or from a situation despite feeling very bored, staring at the television without actually watching it, or suffering from insomnia are indications of poor contact and withdrawal.

The Rhythm of Contact and Withdrawal Is Determined by the Styles of Contact

According to the Gestalt approach, the rhythm of contact and withdrawal is determined by the ways the person uses to establish contact with his/her environment, or in other words, by his/her contact styles. Perls et al. (1951/1996) stated that people use six different contact styles in interpersonal relations and named them introjection, confluence, projection, retroflection, desensitization, and egotism. Later, Polster and Polster (1974, 89) added "deflection" as another contact style, and Crocker (1981) drew attention to a different form of retroflection and called it proflection. The contact styles that an individual uses while interacting with others are explained in detail in the upcoming sections. However, in order to get an idea about them, they are briefly explained below by using the metaphor of eating, which is widely used in the Gestalt approach.

Introjection. It means that the person accepts all those sensations, thoughts, and behaviors that come from the environment, "as it is," without discriminating and absorbing. An introjecting person is one who swallows without chewing.

Desensitization. It means that the person is not aware of the sensations and feelings that come from his/her body. A desensitized person eats without being aware of the taste and smell of the food.

Deflection. It means that the person does not see or hear the messages, reactions, and emotional expressions of other people. A deflecting person shuts his/her mouth tightly to avoid eating.

Projection. It means that the person attributes his/her own emotions, thoughts, behaviors, or characteristics to another person, situation, or object. A projecting person either spits out or vomits whatever he/she eats.

Retroflection. It means that the person shows what he/she expects (such as love, attention, anger) from others to his/her self or to others. A retroflected person either bites his/her own lips instead of eating, or he/she does not eat but feeds other people.

Egotism. It means that the person is watching him/herself as an outside observer. The person seems to like watching him/herself in the mirror while eating.

Confluence. It means that the person sees him/herself and others as being a "single entity" and cannot define his/her own boundaries. A confluent person eats only when the other person eats and expects the other person do the same.

Clarkson (1991, 50) represented these contact styles in a diagram as follows:

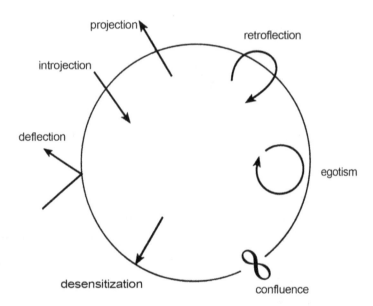

The individual uses these aforementioned contact styles in order to satisfy his/her needs from the environment. If the styles of contact the individual uses helps him/her to actualize his/her desires and needs, then the gestalt is completed and the individual withdraws for a while.

In other words, the rhythm of contact and withdrawal is not disrupted. If the style of contact the individual uses does not help or even prevents him/her from actualizing his/her desires and needs, then the gestalt is not completed and the contact-withdrawal rhythm is disrupted. In the Gestalt approach, the styles of contact that prevent the individual from satisfying his/her needs are placed under the headings "contact disorders," "interruptions to contact," "boundary disturbances," "resistances," and "dysfunctional contact styles." As can be seen, these expressions have "negative" connotations and give an impression that all these contact styles are harmful or disadvantegous; they should thus not be used. However, it is not the style of contact itself but when, how, toward whom, in which situation, how frequently, and for how long these contact styles are used that cause the "disorder," "interruption," "disturbance," "resistance," or "dysfunction." In other words, the contact styles are neither beneficial nor harmful per se. Whether they are beneficial or harmful is determined by the conditions in which they are used. For this reason, in this book, the phrase "contact styles" is preferred to the aforementioned expressions, and both advantages and disadvantages of using these contact styles are explained with examples in the relevant sections.

While establishing contact with the environment, it is possible to use the contact styles independently from each other or in various combinations. For example, introjection takes place on the basis of all the other contact styles and therefore accompanies them without exception. In some instances, the person might use the contact styles in such a complicated way that it becomes difficult to understand which styles of contact are used or to differentiate the styles from each other. Contact styles hold a very important place in the Gestalt approach because understanding how and in which ways the person is interrupting the satisfaction of his/her needs contributes a lot to the determination of what to work on and how in therapy. Hence, in Gestalt therapy, contact styles are one of the most important maps that show the way to the therapist. Information regarding how this map can be used in therapy is given in the chapter entitled "A Case Presentation."

Both the Individual and the Environment Are Equally Responsible for Disrupting the Rhythm of Contact and Withdrawal

According to the Gestalt approach, both the individual and the environment are equally responsible for disrupting the rhythm of contact and withdrawal, or in other words, they are equally responsible for not being able to find a balance or to establish a harmony between them (Perls 1973, 16). Thus, it is not right to blame solely the individual or the environment for the disharmony between them. For instance, our behaviors play as much a role as our partner's behaviors in the deterioration of our relations. As the problem was created by both parties, they must work on the solution to the problem together and take equal responsibility for resolving it.

The most fundamental reason for disruption of the balance is the differentiation of the needs of the individual and the needs of the society and the inability of the person to distinguish whether his/her needs or those of society are more important (Perls 1973, 28). Every group that is formed by individuals who are in a functional relation to one another, such as a family, school, city, or country can be accepted as "society." Because of the need to establish contact with other human beings, the individual has a tendency to establish contact with the "society" to which he/she feels he/she belongs. However, during contact, sometimes conflicts may arise between the needs of the individual and the needs of society or the needs of other individuals in the group. If such conflict does emerge, the individual is obliged to decide which one of his/her needs has the paramount importance, and according to his/her decision, he/she either chooses to maintain the contact or to withdraw. In either case, the person gives up that need that he/she has decided is less important, but this does not cause much nuisance to the person or the society. However, if the person spends a long time in deciding or is dissatisfied with the choice he/she has made, he/she can neither establish good contact nor withdraw. This situation creates a nuisance for both the individual and the society. The person may tend to choose one of two unhealthy ways when he/she is unable to make a choice between his/her needs or is not satisfied with his/her choices. One of the unhealthy ways is crossing the boundaries of the society and, instead of withdrawing, violating the rules of the society and putting oneself in the position of an offender. A person who commits offense cannot distinguish the boundaries between him/herself and the others and thus cannot perceive or understand the needs of others. The other unhealthy way is to withdraw excessively and to allow society to violate one's boundaries. In this case, the person becomes neurotic. The neurotic, just like the offender, cannot distinguish the boundaries between him/herself and the others; however, in contrast to the offender, the neurotic is unaware of his/her own needs. Whilst a neurotic gives more importance to society than him/herself, an offender, on the contrary, gives more importance to him/herself than society. Healthy individuals, on the other hand, neither allow society to violate their boundaries nor violate the boundaries of the society.

In short, different from other approaches that believe that the disruption of the balance between the individual and environment arises solely from the individual or the environment, the Gestalt approach focuses on the disorders emerging on the "contact boundary" between the person and the environment rather than focusing on the disorders of the person or the disorders of society. Therefore, the characteristics of the contact boundary, as well as the contact-withdrawal rhythm, are examined carefully during therapy. One of the tasks of the therapist is to help the client to create the most appropriate and best rhythm for him/herself.

8

INTROJECTION

What Is Introjection?

The introjection style of contact forms the basis of all other contact styles. A newborn baby, in addition to basic needs such as air, food, and water, needs the attention, love, and guidance of those who are taking care of him/her in order to survive, grow, and develop. The things that will satisfy these needs have to be offered to and received by the baby. In the beginning, as the baby's capacity is very limited, he/she introjects wholly whatever is offered and has no chance to choose. For example, before teething occurs, the baby swallows milk as it is by sucking, with no need to bite or chew. In a similar way, the baby accepts the love, attention, or anger shown by those around as they are. In other words, the baby—as a passive receiver—introjects everything that is offered as it is, without making any choices, distinctions, controls, and arrangements. When newly born, babies have no knowledge. From the moment of birth on, they start receiving information about themselves, the world, what is good, or what is bad primarily from parents and other people around. Since their intellectual capacity is limited and as they are inexperienced, the babies accept all this information, all these attitudes and manners, without thinking or questioning, and accept them all as if they are right. In the Gestalt approach, this is called introjection. In other words, introjection is accepting and swallowing any message from the environment as it is (Perls et al. 1951/1996, 199).

Later, the situation changes when the baby teethes and passes on to solid food. The baby now has to divide the food into small pieces, chew them, and get them ready for digestion before swallowing them. If this does not happen, the food cannot be digested, and various digestion problems emerge. The baby, and later the child, either tries to throw the food out, that is, vomits, or if it is not possible, the baby/child becomes poisoned, has stomachache or cramps, and thus becomes sick. In other words, when externally received food is presented in a form that is appropriate for the needs and the structure of the organism, they contribute to its growth and development, while food that is inappropriate to the needs and structure of the organism destroys its physiological health. The same is also true for psychological well being. That is, as the baby grows, as his/her intellectual capacity and experiences increase, he/she should question the information and messages related to him/her, the others and the environment, should examine them, should accept those that are appropriate, and should either change the inappropriate ones to fit him/her or reject them completely. Otherwise, just like the inappropriate food poisoning or sickening the baby, what is introjected will poison and make him/her sick, unhappy, and will damage his/her psychological health. The adaption of external information to the individual's needs after evaluation is called assimilation (Perls et al. 1951/1996, 189). In other words, assimilation is the evaluation and adaptation of those introjections appropriate for the person. For understanding the difference between introjection and assimilation, the following example can be helpful. Let us assume that an individual has learned the message "early to bed, early to rise makes a man healthy, wealthy, and wise." If that person constantly goes to bed and gets up early and is comfortable with it, then he or she has assimilated this message. However if the person feels guilty when not going to bed early or goes to bed early but is bothered by missing the evening hours, then this person has introjected the message as it is, that is, he/she has not assimilated it. According to Perls et al. (1951/1996, 189), while assimilation helps the growth and development of personality introjection obstructs them.

One of the examples that can be given for introjection is learning to talk. It is clear that one of the best ways of learning is through imitation and modeling. Starting from the first day of his/her life, the child hears the voices of those around and eventually recognizes the specific meaning of these voices. Then, when ready, he/she starts introjecting the same sounds by imitating. In time the child learns the corresponding meanings of the sounds and properly starts talking. Some children introject not only the sounds but also the manner of speech. For example, the manners of speech of some mother-daughter or father-son pairs are so much alike that they cannot be distinguished on the phone. Comments such as "She smiles just like her mother" or "He stares just like his father when angry" emphasize certain characteristics introjected from parents.

The messages we have introjected from our environment guide us in making sense of ourselves, our relations, and our lives. There are so many things we have introjected from others—the food we like, our taste in clothes, the type of relations we are seeking, the categorization of the behaviors as good or bad. Some introjections are in the form of "should" (Clarkson 1991, 53). For example, "You should always work," "You should treat your brother nicely," "You should stop at red lights." Some of the introjections are related to social life and culture (Sills et al. 1998, 61). For example, "Don't talk unless you are asked," "When you visit somebody's home, do not sit before you are offered a seat," "When the national anthem plays, stand up and keep still." There are yet other introjections that are related to prejudices and clichés (Fantz 1998, 120), such as "Men are rude," "Women are weak," and "Time is money." Another type is totally introjecting a certain person, such as one's mother or father (Perls 1969/1996). In such cases, the parent who is introjected is generally not the most loved one, but the parent who is powerful and in control. It is also possible to introject not all but some personality traits of the parents.

Psychologically the most important introjected messages are those related to ourselves such as "You are very lazy," "You are more creative than your brother," or "You are so sensitive." This type of messages can be introjected not only as voiced statements but also by watching, observing, or feeling (Daş 2002). For example, if, even when a child does something good or brings home a very good school report, the parents do not give any feedback or react with "Well, this is how it should be anyway," then the child could reach the conclusion that "no matter what I do, it will not be worth talking about. I am obviously an insignificant person who cannot do anything worthwhile." A child who realizes that sexual subjects are never mentioned at home might think that "since it is never mentioned, then sexuality must be a very shameful and bad thing." When a child talks, if nobody looks at him/her, then he/she may develop such an introjection as "They don't pay attention to what I am saying. I must be very stupid." Such introjected information can guide a person's whole life. For example, a person who has introjected that he/she is stupid generally chooses one of the following two paths. The first path is to accept being "stupid" and to constantly sabotage him/herself on the basis of this knowledge and thus turn him/herself into a failure. These individuals, by not concentrating, being very anxious, not working, abusing alcohol or drugs, wasting their time and money, or engaging in unrequited love relations, condemn themselves to failure and act as if they are broadcasting their "stupidity" to the whole world. The second path is refusing to accept "being stupid" and trying to prove to everybody how intelligent he/she is. In contrast to the former, these are perfectionist individuals who are constantly striving for success. They try to be the best, the most hard working, most knowledgeable, most beautiful, the slimmest, the best talker, and the cleanest person, and no matter how high their performance is, they are never pleased with themselves because deep down, they actually believe that they are stupid.

> *While reading these lines, are you becoming aware of certain messages you have introjected? For example, what could be your message about getting help? Is it "Never bother people by asking for help unless absolutely necessary"? Is it "Do everything yourself, never ask for help? Is it "Ask for help, there is always someone who can help you"? Or is it "Even if I ask for help, they will not help anyway"? Is it "I can't do anything without getting help"? Or is it something else? Which is your introjected message? Or is it assimilated?*

The Advantages and Disadvantages of Introjection

Introjection, since it is based on learning, is beneficial in matters such as talking, reading-writing, or learning a foreign language. It is also helpful when learning to drive or how to use a tool, to develop therapy skills, or to design a building. Similarly, when a student is studying the night before the exam, to accept the knowledge without questioning is good in terms of being successful in that exam. As can be seen from all these examples, introjection is advantageous in cases of knowledge previously discovered and developed by other people. It is useless to rediscover such knowledge from scratch. Similarly, we do not need to re-create traffic rules, rules of etiquette, or basic social rules, and their introjection makes our daily lives much easier. Such introjected information enables the integration of the individual into the society (Polster 1995, 32). In some cases, the introjected information may not be so important for us. For example, if my son tells me that X is a good football team, and if this is not an important issue for me, there is no need for me to inquire further or question the issue. I can easily introject "X as a good team" and thus can enjoy watching their games with my son. Yontef (1993, 213) has indicated that introjection can be useful for those individuals who lack the developmental maturity and support to confront their environmental pressures.

According to Perls (1973, 34), introjection can be dangerous in two ways. The first is the failure of a person to establish and to develop his/her personality as he/she constantly tries to wholly include the values, concepts, attitudes, and habits coming from his/her environment within his/her system. In such cases, introjection overloads the person, giving him/her no chance for self-discovery. Introjection turns the person into a waste basket of extraneous and irrelevant information (Perls 1973, 34). Introjection makes us something like a house so jampacked with other people's possessions that there is no room for the owner's property (Clarkson and Mackewn 1993, 73). The second type of danger caused by introjection is the obstruction of the integration of the personality. Introjecting two completely opposite values, attitudes, or concepts can be an example of this. When two contrasting maxims such as "Do not do to others what you do not want done to you" and "In order to succeed in life, ruthless competition is a must" are introjected, then it is not easy for that person to integrate these two points of view since according to the former one needs to be polite, calm, and gentle, while according to the latter, one should be insistent, contentious, and tough. Consequently, the person is split between them and cannot integrate.

Clarkson (1991, 53) has pointed out that introjection prevents the mobilization of the person and the appropriate satisfaction of his/her needs. The reason for the prevention of mobilization is the disharmony between the wishes and needs of that person and what he/she is introjected. For example, a girl who has introjected the information that "Men are evil" will not be able to get close to a man, even when she is attracted to him. A woman who has introjected the notion that "A good mother should always be with her children and should not be interested in anything else" will not be able to fulfill her career ambitions and will remain a housewife. In such cases, even if the person is not aware of it, his/her wishes still prevail and they remain as unfinished business to be satisfied sometime in the future. Perls et al. (1951/1996, 190) stated that the introjections that prevent the completion of an act diminish the person's enthusiasm and life energy and can even completely destroy them. The introjecting individuals, by spending part of their life energy on the repression and forgetting of their original desires, are actually fighting with themselves (Clarkson and Mackewn 1993, 72). The person who is under the influence of what he/she has introjected feels an internal pressure to behave according to what is introjected and, when acting or even thinking to the contrary, feels uncomfortable (Joyce and Sills 2003, 125).

Shub (1998a, 6) divides introjection into two as positive and negative. Here, these terms do not indicate whether or not what is introjected is "good" or "bad" but are used in the context of to what extent the introjected beliefs obstruct or facilitate the person's contact with the environment. In other words, when the person's contact with the environment is obstructed, we are talking about a negative introjection, and when contact is made easily, then we talk about positive introjection. Hence, in terms of deterioration of psychological health, it is not the positive but the negative introjections that are significant. Negative introjections, by obstructing the contact of the person, cause suffering, loss of self-confidence, and thus limit his/her freedom, creativity, and vitality.

Yontef (1993, 495) stated that introjection could lead to feelings of extreme guilt and shame. He pointed out that frequent use of the introjection style of contact would lead to extensive tensions in the areas of the mouth and jaw, the throat and base of the skull, the chest and upper back and the diaphragm. Introjections also play a part in eating disorders and alcohol dependency.

The Basis of Introjection

Polster (1995, 32–37) explains the introjection process via the concept of the "introjection triad" that consists of (a) contact, (b) configuration, and (c) tailoring. According to this model, in order to introject something the person has to have contact with the world. This contact provides the "raw material" of introjection. The second stage of introjection process is configuration. Initially what is introjected is organized very loosely and becomes stable only over time. The discord between the needs of the child and what the family provides makes the configuration—that is, the organization of what will be introjected—more difficult. For example, a delay in the serving of food even despite the child's obvious hunger, suppression by the parents of the child's aggressive instinct, putting of a distance when the child wants to be close to others, the father's insulting attitude when the child is generous to his or her friends, or being called stupid in a household where success is deemed very important are cases where great difficulty is encountered in configuration. Through tailoring the early experiences, which are first organized very weakly, in time become the basis of the personality and turn into rigid and repetitive behaviors (Yontef 1993, 183)

The formation of introjection requires two conditions. The first of these is that the information to be introjected must be repeated frequently, and the second, the information must be emotion loaded, that is, while introjecting the information the person must experience intense feelings (Shub 1998a, 8). For example, if a little girl who wants to do something by herself or to discover things around her often receives messages such as "You are too young, you can't do it" or "You are a girl, you can't go alone" and when she insists and resists is scolded or punished, then she would naturally feel bad. Similarly, a child who receives messages such as "Crying doesn't suit you at all," "Those who cry are weak," or "Nobody likes you when you cry" every time he or she cries will inevitably feel even more sad. Since one of the most basic psychological needs of a child is to receive the love, approval, and admiration of his or her family, in time the child foregoes the meeting of his or her needs and chooses instead to fulfill what the parents want. Thus, the child eventually becomes an adult who has difficulty in deciding by him/herself, who feels very anxious whenever he/she has to do something on his/her own and who never cries. Even though what we have introjected generally comes from our childhood years when we are most fragile and most impressionable and is learned from those we most love, it can also be learned in the later periods of our lives from many sources in our environment whether close to us or not. For example, friends, lovers, teachers, colleagues, artists, and even television programs can be the determinants of what we are going to introject.

Kepner (1987, 175) likens a child to a vulnerable house with all its windows open located in the middle of a plain with no trees around. This is such a situation that should a wind blow, that is, if the adults intervene contrary to the desires and needs of the child, everything in the house may be blown out or just the opposite could happen and things from the outside may easily get into the house. In such cases, that is, in families where there is a great deal of intervention with the boundaries of the child, the child generally chose one of two paths. The first is to give up on him/herself for the sake of his/her family. Here, the child forgets his own desires and needs in order to meet those of his/her family. The second path is to totally close oneself off to the outside. In some cases the child closes off him/herself to such an extent that he/she does not introject anything coming from the family.

Personality Characteristics of People Who Use Introjection as a Contact Style Frequently

People who use introjection as a style of contact frequently, instead of questioning or expressing themselves, prefer to comply with the rules.

Even when accused by others, they do not object, do not answer, do not explain, and do not demand an explanation. Introjection makes the person lazy. On the other hand to question something and to discuss it requires a considerable amount of energy and time. Such people are impatient, they want solutions to be offered in a liquid form and pre-prepared so that they can immediately swallow them when necessary (Perls et al. 1951/1996, 328). As they prefer to hold what they have swallowed as a whole in their stomach instead of biting, chewing, and digesting, even if they are not happy with them, they continue with their existing situations and relations. They focus on adverse possibilities in case of a change in the status quo and ignore the positive possibilities. For such individuals, even to start a new job, to buy something new, or to move to a new place could be very difficult (Zinker 1994, 122).

Introjecting people can be easily influenced by authority figures. They act according to what others want them to do and take on the responsibility of things that are not their business at all (Smith 1977, 15). They cannot act creatively, spontaneously, or with foresight in their work (Zinker 1994, 126). They are so involved with what they should do that, when asked what they want, can hardly answer because they are not aware of their own needs. They cannot regulate or manage their lives according to their needs.

In families where introjects dominate, the energy level is low. Such families prefer to carry out things in the traditional ways and to behave according to the old rules. They do not bother with producing new and creative solutions. In these families, generally, a member imposes an idea or a solution on the others, and they accept it wholly, without questioning. Active discussions cannot be seen in such families. This, while leading to a conjectural sense of security, also leads to artificial agreements where nothing is actually solved. The decisions of such families are not taken according to their specific conditions but always according to generally accepted rules (McConville 1995, 142–143).

How to Work with Introjection in Therapy

The purpose of introjection work in therapy is to make the client aware of what he/she introjected, to have him/her question them, to work on them until they are relevant for that person, and to assimilate the new knowledge. To become aware of what is introjected and to change it is a difficult process that requires much effort and time. Some preparatory steps are necessary in order to start working on introjections during therapy (Shub 1998a).

These are:

a. Exploring the background of the client and how the introjection process has developed

b. Helping the client to be aware of his or her inner processes and the contact styles he/she used to interrupt contact

c. Informing the client about the introjection process.

Once the preparations are completed, the first thing to do is to help the client to become aware of his/her introjections. For this, the therapist can use various questions based on the expressions the client typically uses. For example Gloria, who had been attending therapy for some time, mentioned how that morning because she had many things to do, asked her sister to iron her slacks, but then how annoyed she was thinking that her sister would be tired when ironing them and she didn't want to tire her unnecessarily." Then work was started on the meaning behind the use of "unnecessary," and eventually it was found that the thought of "I am such a worthless person that it is not even worth the time and effort of another person to press my slacks" was lying behind it. When an introjected message is reached during therapy, then the therapist should start investigating how and from whom that message was learned and how it has affected the client's life. For example, when working with Gloria, investigations were carried out into the answers to questions such as how she knew that she was worthless, what her memories were that suggested that she was worthless, at which times she felt worthless, whether she really saw herself as worthless, what being worthless meant to her, and how believing herself to be worthless was affecting her life.

For some clients, it is easier to find a connection between what is introjected and how and from whom these introjections were learned. On the other hand, some clients find it very difficult to find any connection between their introjected beliefs and their past lives. Difficulty in finding a connection generally appears in cases where introjections have led to too much pain and have been experienced in a very dramatic way. The greater the emotional load related with the introjection

- The more difficult it is for the introjected message to surface,
- The more powerful the introjected message is,
- The more the contact is interfered with by the introjected message,
- The more difficult it is to change the introjected message (Shub 1998a, 18).

Shub (1998a, 32) has suggested that in cases where it is difficult to find a connection between from whom and how the introjected message has been learned, preparing a map with the client can be very helpful. When preparing the map, the client might be asked to list the significant people in his/her life, starting from childhood. Then time is spent on the importance of these people on the client's life, their distinct personality traits, and the client's relation with them. For example, following the work carried out by Tess, who had introjected the message "I am stupid" but who could not find the connections from whom and how she learned it, the following map was prepared:

Map of Negative Introjections

Mother: *A loving, docile housewife, not too caring toward Tess, is not much interested in her schoolwork; she doesn't want her to get an education but to get married and have children.*

Father: *He is not home much; when at home, more interested in her brother; he is proud when she does something good but takes the credit on himself, saying, "Eh, whose daughter are you?" or "If it wasn't for me, you couldn't have done this."*

Grandfather: *Gives great importance to being clever but believes that girls cannot be very clever and hence is forgiving to her faults, does not get angry with her, loves her.*

Primary school teacher:	*Likes her, says she is a good kid but makes* her sit her at the back of the class and does not ask her to perform in the class very often.

During the work carried out on this map, it was understood that Tess perceived her mother's indifferent attitude toward her and her mother's wish for her to marry as meaning "I am not smart enough to have an education and to be cared for." She interpreted her grandfather's tolerance toward her mistakes as meaning "Poor girl, she doesn't know anything anyway, better I don't push her." Tess evaluated her father's greater attention to her brother as suggesting "As you are a girl you are unimportant" and saw her primary school teacher's behavior as labeling her as "A stupid but good girl, best not call upon in the class so as not to make a fool of her."

During therapy, one of the ways to make the clients fully aware of their introjected messages and to have them to articulate their feelings and thoughts related to these messages more clearly is to ask them to exaggerate the introjected message as much as possible. For example, the client might be asked to express his or her feelings regarding perceived worthlessness in an exaggerated way by starting, "I am so worthless that I have no value whatsoever," and later work can be carried out on this. Another practice could be to start a dialogue between the introjected message and its exact opposite in two-chair work. The client, for example, might be asked to establish a dialogue between "I am worthless" and "I am valuable" or "I am stupid" and "I am smart." In this practice, the client when sitting on one of the chairs talks according to the introjected message—"worthless" or "stupid"—and when on the other, talks for the other side—"valuable" or "smart." In this way it will be possible for the client to experience and review these opposing messages and to integrate them within the self.

Another two-chair experiment that can be used in therapy is to have the client set up a dialogue with the person who taught him or her that message. In this practice, the client talks as him/herself when sitting on one chair and as the other person when on the other. For example, as mentioned above, Tess, who has introjected the message "I am stupid" told her grandfather that she was very pleased that he loved her and was tolerant toward her, but she was very sorry and angry to see that he did not think that girls could be smart. After she explained how these two attitudes played a role in her feeling stupid, she moved to her grandfather's place and voiced his feelings and thoughts after hearing what she had said. Then, moving once again to her place, she continued to talk about her own feelings and thoughts. The purpose of such a practice is to enable the clients to express their feelings about the introjected message to the other person, to be aware of the feelings and thoughts of the other person who taught them that message, and to experience a healthier way of making contact with that person while protecting themselves.

While working with introjections, another significant practice that can be carried out is the empty chair technique. In this practice, the client is asked to give back the introjected message to its owner—i.e., the person who taught it—and explains the new message he/she has developed. For example, during such work carried out with Tess, she first set her mother in the other chair and told her what she was feeling because of her careless attitude toward her and her lack of interest in her schoolwork. During this, Tess experienced a deep sorrow and intense anger. Later, she gave back to her mother the message "I am stupid" by saying, "It is your idea, your truth," and concluded the correct message to be "I am not stupid at all, I am even clever, I have had many successes, and even if you do not see them, I can see them now." Since such experiments can reveal very intense feelings, the therapist has to be highly skilled in working with such feelings.

One of the techniques frequently applied in the Gestalt approach is language work. Applications that involve changing the language used are very useful, particularly when working with introjections. This can be carried out by changing expressions in the form of "should" or "must" into "I want," "I choose," or "I prefer." For example, the client can be asked to change "I shouldn't be angry with him" into "I choose not to be angry with him," "I must study hard" into "I want to study hard" or "I must go there" into "I prefer to go there." Language experiments can also be used in changing the client's expressions regarding him/herself. For example, "I think I am stupid" can be changed into "I prefer to think that I am stupid" or "I am lazy" into "I want to believe that I am lazy."

The purpose of such work is to have the person take responsibility for what he or she says.

In some cases, what are preventing the contact are not the introjected negative messages but positive messages that have not been assimilated. A person with few positive introjections looks like a box from which the bottom has been cut out, so each time a positive comment is put in the box, it passes straight through and falls to the ground; the box is never filled. Actually, assimilated positive messages play a very significant role in the development of self-respect and self-esteem. Hence, another theme that should be emphasized during therapy is the development and reinforcement of such positive messages. The work on development and reinforcement of positive messages goes through the following stages (Daş 2003b).

Evaluation of Positive Messages

At this stage, the therapist tries to gather information on areas such as the client's level of self-respect and self-esteem, the positive thoughts of the client concerning him/herself, how the client copes with difficult situations, and how the client makes contact with people.

Identification of Positive Characteristics

During this period of work, the therapist gives feedback to the client about those positive characteristics observed by him/her during the sessions. Meanwhile, a list is prepared containing the positive thoughts of the therapist, other related people, and of course, the client concerning him/herself.

Collecting Proof

In order to find proofs related to the positive traits of the client, the first step is to question how convinced the client is about the positive comments of the therapist and other people. At this stage, to enable the client to be more aware of his or her positive characteristics and to strengthen the relevant proofs, client's photographs, school yearbook, letters received, and the like can be used. Furthermore, empty or two-chair practices are very useful here. In the empty-chair work, the client

135

chooses one of the people who had positive opinions about him/herself and, acting as that person, talks with him/herself sitting in the empty chair, explaining what he/she considers being positive features in the client. During the two-chair experiment, on the other hand, the client sets up a dialogue between him/herself and one of the people with positive feelings and thoughts about him/herself. One other method that can be employed in discovering proofs is preparing a Map of Positive Characteristics together with the client. This map is prepared as with the Map of Negative Introjections, but here the focus is on positive traits. While preparing the map, the clients are asked to start from childhood and list people who had a good relationship with them, whom they liked and appreciated. Later, the importance of that person in the client's life, their distinctive character traits, and their positive opinions about the client are added to the list.

Finding the connections with the experiences

The purpose of these practices is to enable the person to find connections with his/her positive characteristics and experiences and help the client in reinforcing his/her belief in his/her positive traits. For this, the situations where the positive traits emerge in the client's existing life can be determined or the possible future situations where the characteristics may surface can be experienced through imagination techniques. At this stage, focusing on what the client is feeling when or in whatever situation his/her positive characteristics are apparent is helpful in the reinforcement of positive emotions.

Assimilation

The assimilation of the defined positive characteristics is a long process. Various experiments can be carried out to ensure that the client does not lose his/her belief in his/her positive traits even in difficult or adverse situations. During this work, besides techniques of imagination, other creative applications such as defining specific body postures for each characteristic, finding objects that represent each of them, or drawing pictures of the situations where these characteristics emerge can be utilized.

In conclusion, as the introjection contact style is the basis of other contact styles, changing introjections is both a very deep and intense work and a very important one as the changes occurring here lead to marked changes in other styles of contact. During such work, the clients face both positive and negative childhood memories, connect them with their current lives, return the introjected "poisonous" information to its owners, and are in a way reborn with new information that is both correct and appropriate for them.

9

DESENSITIZATION

What Is Desensitization?

In its most general sense, desensitization is the numbing of sensations. Desensitization is the ignoring of sensations coming from the body, such as pain or discomfort, and the blocking out of information coming from the environment (Clarkson 1991, 46). It appears in two forms: the first is desensitization to bodily sensations and the other desensitization to emotions.

In physical desensitization, the person is unaware of sensations of seeing, hearing, tasting, smelling, touching, or various combinations of these and feels nothing related to them. Since the person feels nothing, he/she has no response to most of the inner or external stimuli (Sills et al. 1998, 57). A person can even become desensitized to basic needs such as hunger or tiredness. Those who are proud of how much they can drink, how long they can manage to go without sleep, or how they can work for long hours under very hard conditions are actually desensitized to their bodily needs. For the sake of tanning and looking beautiful, lying in the sun for hours with no concern for the adverse effects of the sun light on the skin can be an another example of desensitization. When you have your meal in front of the television, you are again desensitized to your senses because you can neither fully taste what you are eating nor be aware of whether or not you have already eaten enough. Sometimes we suddenly realize that we have lost or gained weight or there are bruises on our arms or legs, but we become aware of this only after it has happened. These are all examples of desensitization.

Are you, while reading this book, desensitized to any of your physical sensations? Maybe you are hungry, thirsty, or maybe your arm is numb, maybe you are sleepy; possibly you are sitting or lying in an uncomfortable position. If any of these applies, please avoid desensitization and care for your body.

According to Kepner (1987, 100), selective-attention, interference with breathing, and chronic muscular contractions play a part in the appearance of desensitization. For example, if a person, either just before or as soon as a sensation becomes apparent, diverts his/her attention to something else through selective perception, then that person is desensitized toward the sensation coming from his/her body. Again, frequent and shallow breathing, or holding the breath prevent the person from being aware of his/her sensations and lead to desensitization. In some cases, desensitization is due to chronic contracting of the muscles. These contractions cause the person to feel nothing in those areas, or to feel either numbness or pins and needles. For example, a chronic contraction may occur in the pelvic region of a person who has sex-related conflicts, and this may cause him/her not to feel anything in that area and consequently effect his/her sexual functions. On the other hand, according to the Gestalt approach, which considers the individual as an integrated whole of body, feelings, and thoughts, desensitization of the person to his/her body might indicate that the person is alienated from some of his/her feelings or some parts of his/her self (Kepner 1987, 97).

In emotional desensitization, in order to be able to cope with the feelings that were caused by negative experiences, the person tries simply not to feel them or in other words desensitize themselves to these feelings. According to Kepner (1982) in desensitization, as a result of dulling of the sensations the background becomes distorted and unrecognizable. Thus as the person becomes desensitized toward his/her sensations, then he/she starts misinterpreting them. For example as seen in the eating disorder bulimia, when the person feels anxiety, he/she interprets this as being hungry and turns to eating. Similarly, alcoholics interpret feelings of anxiety, loneliness, or depressive feelings as a craving for alcohol since they are desensitized to these emotions (Clarkson 1991, 76). On the other hand, becoming desensitized to painful, annoying feelings also causes people to be isolated from the pleasures and joys of life and to become desensitized to them too (Clarkson 1991, 46). Hence, a constant feeling of tiredness, reluctance toward life, or finding life boring or meaningless are also related with desensitization. Another form of desensitization is to focus only on thoughts by intellectualizing everything.

The opposite of desensitization is oversensitivity (Joyce and Sills 2003, 119). Hypochondria can be given as an example of extreme physical over-sensitivity. People suffering from this are constantly on the alert to every sensation of their bodies and show exaggerated reactions to these. People who are in a state of emotional oversensitivity can easily be offended, touchy, or fragile, as they are affected by every stimulus.

The Advantages and Disadvantages of Desensitization

Desensitization when used consciously and occasionally is beneficial and even necessary. For example, desensitization is beneficial in cases of an athlete ignoring the slight pain in his/her foot in order to win the race, a person tolerating an uncomfortable bed in order to be able to sleep, or a student enduring sleeplessness when preparing for an exam. Also, when you have a toothache, to desensitize against the pain until you can find a dentist may be necessary, as may be the case, to desensitize against hunger when you diet. Right now, my desensitization to the loud music coming from my neighbor is advantageous in terms of my being able to continue writing this book. Painkillers, anesthesia, and sleeping pills also give comfort to a person by creating desensitization. However, Perls et al. (1951/1996, 30) point out that as pain, hurt, and insomnia are actually related to retroflection contact style, they need to be investigated.

Desensitization can lead a person to self-harming behavior (Clarkson 1991, 61). First of all, the obstruction of the satisfaction of the basic needs of a person such as hunger and thirst, immobilization, or sleep deprivation for long periods can cause a deterioration in his/her physical health. On the other hand, those people who have become extremely desensitized to hurt and pain, may cut themselves with razors, burn themselves with cigarettes, or bang their heads on the wall until they bleed just for the sake of feeling something; this is undoubtedly both hazardous and undesirable. Again, extreme consumption of alcohol, use of narcotics or stimulants, in order to desensitize or to reverse desensitized sensations is very harmful. Since desensitization prevents pleasure as well as pain, it can cause the person to take high risks such as gambling, frequent one-night stands, or exaggerated sexual experiences in order to be able to feel excitement and pleasure. One of the most important problems arising from desensitization is a feeling of emptiness. Since the person does not know how to fill this void, he/she eventually starts not to enjoy life, to get away from his/her environment, and to become introvert. An overdose of desensitization can lead to loss of self and sense of disembodiment (Kepner 1987, 98). The desensitization style of contact is used frequently in schizoid (Clarkson 1991, 46) and borderline personality disorders (Kepner 1987, 107). This style of contact can be seen in various disorders ranging from unawareness of certain bodily sensations to states of catatonia where the person is not aware of any internal or external stimuli or to stupor, which is observed in cases of severe depression.

The items related with emotional desensitization on the Gestalt Contact Styles Questionnaire (Revised), which was confirmed as reliable and valid by Aktaş and Daş (2002), are given below. Would you like to mark the items and find out how often you use the desensitization type of contact? While answering, after reading each item, circle the letter which best reflects your status. The meaning of each letter is as follows:

A: Highly appropriate for me
B: Appropriate for me
C: I am undecided
D: Not appropriate for me
E: Not appropriate for me at all

1. I sob when I am really sad.	A B C D E
2. My feelings are not easily hurt.	A B C D E

3. I can keep my cool, even in the worst situations. A B C D E

4. I define myself as rational rather than emotional. A B C D E

5. People say that I am an emotional person.   A B C D E

6. I think I am a sensitive person.   A B C D E

The scores of the items are A=1, B=2, C=3, D=4, E=5. Only in items 1, 4 and 5 is reverse scoring used. That is, for those items the scoring is thus: A=5, B=4, C=3, D=2 and E=1. The maximum score you can get from these items is 30. The higher your score, the more you are using desensitization as a style of contact.

The Basis of Desensitization

According to Kepner (1987, 99), disturbance of sensations lies on the basis of the desensitization. Sensations can be disturbing for three basic reasons. The first is the case where sensations unbearably bother the person. Sensations such as pain, hunger, thirst, or cold when experienced deeply or for a long time, both threaten our lives and are very difficult to endure. In those situations, the person tries to tolerate and survive by feeling nothing. For example, during earthquakes, many people who are trapped under the rubble manage to survive the physical pains they experience by desensitization. The second cause is the failure to satisfy the needs. When the needs cannot be met because of various reasons they lead to uncomfortable sensations. For instance, when we are in need of others but cannot find anybody around us or when we are unable to see our family because of the demands of work or school, even though we miss them very much, we might choose the path of desensitization in order to tolerate the feelings of loneliness or longing. The third cause is the conflict between sensations and learned beliefs, or in Gestalt terms, "introjections." For example, being aware of sexual sensations if sexuality is regarded as "bad" or "shameful"; being aware of sadness if the expression of sorrow is seen as "weakness"; or becoming aware of anger against the parents if it is believed that "one does not get mad at parents" become intolerable for the person. So the person desensitizes him/herself to these feelings in order to alleviate the discomfort he/she is experiencing.

Long-term desensitization to bothersome sensations and feelings, while causing the person to lose his/her vitality and feelings also leads him/her to become desensitized to his/her pleasure-giving sensations (Kepner 1987, 100).

In general, there are highly traumatic experiences at the roots of desensitization (Joyce and Sills 2003, 118). For example, Kate talked about witnessing violent fights between her father and mother, how she, along with her siblings and their mother, were beaten during these fights, how during one of the fights her father wounded her mother with a bread knife after which her mother left home, how she and her two siblings had to live with their father after this, how their father would sometimes not come home for two or three days, and there would be neither money nor food in the house during that time, and how her father, who had a very bad temper, once broke two of her fingers because she could not stop the crying of her three-year-old brother. In order to endure these traumatic experiences, Kate had to desensitize herself, and this affected her life in many ways. For example, Kate was extremely overweight because in order not to feel the anxiety and anger she experienced in her traumatic childhood she was desensitized to these feelings and in time she started to interpret these feelings of anxiety and anger as hunger. Hence, every time she became anxious or angry, she would turn to food. There were also razor marks on Kate's arms and legs because she had become desensitized to the hurts in order to stand the physical pains of her childhood beatings. Kate was also desensitized against sadness. The best example of this is her killing her pet bird because it was chirping too much. Kate described her experiences related to this incident like this: "Actually I loved him. I don't know how it happened, but I felt no remorse in killing him and no sorrow afterwards." Children, like Kate, who have had traumatic life experiences, are as if they have buried that undeveloped and fragile child within their desensitized bodies in order to protect themselves from pain, humiliation, and abuse.

Personality Characteristics of People Who Use the Desensitization Contact Style Frequently

Kepner (1982) has stated that individuals who frequently use desensitization as a way of contact have certain characteristic traits. These people complain about numbness, lifelessness, and lack of sensation in various parts of their body. They pay more attention to intellectual activities and experiences than physical ones. They are not aware of their bodily sensations. Instead of paying attention to their bodily sensations when they are under stress or to their physical needs when sick, they ignore them. Just as those who frequently use desensitization as a contact style are desensitized toward their own sensations and feelings, they are also desensitized toward the sensations and feelings of other people. Such people are defined by others as superficial, callous individuals who cannot show empathy.

McConville (1995, 162) has pointed out that the interaction of couples or families that frequently use desensitization as a contact style is stereotypical and lacks emotion. Such families pay little attention to each other, and they do not even fully listen to one another. Contact disappears even before the person has had an opportunity to feel understood (Zinker 1994, 120). They may sometimes have heated arguments but do not expect much from each other because they have already given up the idea of getting what they want. In homes where desensitization is often used, there is a joyless and suffocating atmosphere of boredom. Family members lose themselves in the television. In such families, new ideas and suggestions are not taken seriously. Through desensitization, the members protect both themselves and others from being hurt, and so they feel secure, but this sense of security is highly artificial. Couples who frequently resort to desensitization refrain from touching each other; even if they do touch, it is without any genuine feeling. This is also relevant for their sex life. They are generally apathetic where sex is concerned and cannot reach satisfaction during intercourse.

How to Work with Desensitization in Therapy

While working with desensitization during therapy, the goal is to enable the person to reexperience his/her sensations and feelings. This is a very slow and painful process. It is particularly hard for the person to be motivated for therapy if he/she is experiencing strong feelings of emptiness and confusion. In cases of psychosis or heavy depression, the person must be oriented toward medical help. Symptoms such as stiffness or immobilization of the body, an expressionless face, tension in the facial muscles, holding of the breath, avoidance of a particular subject such as sex, inability to express feelings, difficulty in remembering, or willingness to do something but lack of energy to do it may also be significant indications of desensitization (Frantz 1998, 120). When such symptoms appear during therapy, the therapist should investigate to which sensations and feelings the client is desensitized. Another feature that needs attention in terms of desensitization is the tone of voice and the manner of speech. For example, when the client talks about a very heavy experience such as death, terminal illness, or sexual abuse in a monotonous tone as if giving the weather report or talks about them as if they happened to somebody else, then desensitization should be suspected. Again, for example, when a client twists his/her ankle when entering the room but keeps on walking as if nothing happened or sits in a very uncomfortable position for a long time, whether or not desensitization is involved should be investigated.

When working with desensitization during therapy, the first thing to be done is experiments that lead to body awareness. Here, the purpose is to get the clients' attention away from their thoughts and orient them toward their bodily experiences and thus make those bodily experiences important. For this, the client might to be asked to close his/her eyes and focus on every part of his/her body individually, or he/she can be asked to focus only on a particular part of the body, such as the chest or the belly. This goes together with work on accompanying feelings. Furthermore, experiments that make the client aware of the way he/she is sitting, of slight bodily movements, facial expressions, and the use of the voice can also be helpful. Another type of experiments that can be used while working with desensitization is those that involve touching. Desensitization to body parts is generally related to pain, suffering, and emotional hurt. Because of this, the sensitivity in those parts cannot be understood without touching. Therefore to ask the client to touch different parts of his/her body or, when deemed necessary, to have the therapist touch them could help in revealing the desensitized parts (Kepner 1987, 104). However, before progressing to experiments that involve touching, a complete trust relation should be reached between the client and the therapist. Furthermore, extreme care should be shown in such practices, the client should be asked for permission and should be informed that the exercise can be terminated whenever he/she wants. Another method that can be used to activate physical awareness and sensations could be by movement and dance (Kepner 1987, 104). Here the aim is to express feelings through body language.

Another characteristic worth exploring for recognition of feelings is the manner of breathing. For example, holding the breath prevents the recognition and expression of feelings. Frequent or shallow breathing, rapid or loud exhaling could prevent the recognition of feelings. In such cases, and in other cases where the client is unaware of his/her feelings, the therapist could ask the client, "If you should be feeling something, what could it be?" or "If it was somebody else, what would he/she feel?" or the therapist could talk about his/her own feelings.

While working on the awareness of sensations, feelings such as sorrow, anger, anxiety, fear, and grief can be experienced very intensely. It is crucial that the therapist is sufficiently experienced to deal with such feelings; otherwise it might lead the client to go once more and more deeply into new desensitization. At the end of desensitization reversal work, the clients will be in contact with the traumatic incidents and negative feelings of the past, will have completed their unfinished business, and will have integrated all these into themselves. This gives them a base from which they can move on to pleasure, joy, and happiness with an open-heart and courage.

10

DEFLECTION

What Is Deflection?

Deflection as a style of contact was first mentioned by Polster and Polster (1974, 89), according to whom deflection is the avoidance of direct contact with other people or with objects, situations, and events in the environment; thus, it is a reduction in the density and degree of contact. In this style of contact, the person directs his or her energy in other directions in order to reduce the impact of information coming from the environment and to avoid the strong sensations that could emerge from possible contact; in this way, the person moves away from the target (Sills et al. 1998, 59). In other words, deflection is used to make the stimuli coming from the environment rebound from the contact boundary without affecting us. The purpose of deflection is self-protection in disturbing situations. In this way, by isolating him/herself, the person prevents a comment or an action oriented toward him/her from reaching its target, i.e. him/herself (Philippson 2001, 100).

Deflection can be achieved in many ways. Examples are talking around an issue, talking too much, laughing off a comment, avoiding eye contact, pretending to be listening, giving vague answers instead of specific ones, focusing on details rather than the main subject, giving unrelated examples, or not giving any examples when explaining something, using overly polite or stereotypical language, expressing feelings by alleviating or embellishing them, mentioning the past or the future when the present is important, or diminishing the importance of what is being said by shrugging it off (Polster and Polster 1974, 90). Frequent coughing, yawning, or scratching while someone is talking, talking without a pause, forgetting what one is talking about and thus encouraging a change of subject, making jokes continuously, laughing at inappropriate moments, and talking in great detail or abstractly are also examples of deflection (Fantz 1998, 122–123).

During deflection, both the person who is talking and the one listening feel that they are not able to reach each other or are misunderstood (Korb et al. 1989, 59). For example, when Miriam asked Ted, who was looking dispiritedly out of the window, "What is the matter?" and Ted replied, "Nothing," then Ted was preventing Miriam from asking further questions and also avoiding explaining what was bothering him via deflection. Returning from a long trip, when Nancy said to her mother, "I missed you so much," and her mother answered, "Your hair has grown too long, it looks bad," it is possible to say that Nancy's mother is deflecting. One of the relationships where deflection is used most frequently is that of the husband and wife. For example, women in particular feel the need to ask their spouses quite frequently whether or not they love them. In such a situation, answers such as "Well, as we are married . . ." or "Love is a star beyond the clouds" are deflections. Similarly, after a sad incident between the husband and wife, if the husband asks his crying wife, "What happened? Did your mother bother you again?" then this is another example of deflection. Yet another example is the mother's reply of "Ah, how rude of you to say stupid" to her child who says, "I don't want to play with that stupid kid." Sometimes a person may think that he is talking very clearly but not be aware of the fact that he/she is deflecting. However, if the other person is not able to understand what you are saying, if you are not getting the reaction you are expecting, if he/she is asking, "How did we come to this point?" or if he/she is continuously asking questions, then most probably you are deflecting.

To shake hands using only the tips of fingers, to stand away, or to keep the upper or lower part of the body back, to look down or up while talking to someone may also be considered deflection. To close one's eyes when faced with a terrible scene or to close one's ears against a high-pitched sound are also other examples for deflection. Another way of deflection is to orient a certain feeling or need not to its real target but to another one (Latner 1992, 40). For example while you are actually mad at your boss, to take it out on your child, to be angry with your upstairs neighbors for making noise although it is not late, or to nag your spouse, complaining that "this meal is no good" are also deflections.

We can see from these examples that the deflecting person prefers not to see or hear external stimuli and protects him/herself by trying not to be affected by them. The opposite of deflection is being overly affected by the environment and "taking in" everything (Joyce and Sills 2003, 118). In other words, it is to be open to every stimulus from the environment, to be affected by all of them, and not to be able to protect yourself.

The Advantages and Disadvantages of Deflection

Deflection can be used in both harmful and beneficial ways. In cases where we are not yet ready to deal with a certain situation, deflection can help us in gaining time and enduring the situation (Crocker 1999, 10). For example, when we hear about a serious illness or death of someone close to us, we try through deflection not to believe and accept this news for a while in order to be able to cope with that situation. Children who are constantly witnessing fights between their parents, in order to deal with their feelings of being scared, sadness, and anger, deflect by not mentioning them at all (Clarkson 1991, 52) Again, particularly those who have had a major traffic accident, in order not be accused or face a great loss, might at first not remember the accident and might not even ask questions about it.

Korb et al. (1989, 59) pointed out the frequent use of deflection in the realm of politics, diplomacy, science, and various areas of business through the use of overly polite and stereotypical language and indicated that such conscious deflections could be healthy and functional. For example, even if diplomatic language seems very artificial, it prevents the straining of relations between countries by holding back the countries from demeaning each other and expressing their problems too harshly. Under certain circumstances, it may be advantageous to pretend not to hear what is being said. For example, while arguing with someone you love, even though you are sure that his/her real feelings are not these, the person might have uttered harsh words or said things that could make you very angry or hurt. In such cases, it might be smarter and necessary to deflect and not to take on the anger of the other person (Polster and Polster 1974, 90).

In some other cases, in order to meet a need, it might be necessary temporarily to deflect other needs. For example, while I am writing this book, I am deflecting some of my needs such as chatting with my friends or going for a walk. In certain situations, in order to meet a need, it might be appropriate for a person to focus his/her attention in another direction. For example, to silently sing the songs you know while having your tooth filled or while donating blood can be a healthy use of deflection.

There is no doubt that using deflection as a way of contact constantly and without awareness can lead to serious problems and cause a person to wander away both from him/herself and others and become isolated (Korb et al. 1989, 60). At the same time, deflection prevents a person from getting what he/she wants from life (Clarkson 1991, 81). Deflection causes significant problems in relationships. The person faced with deflection feels pressured, confused, in a void, unloved, insignificant, and demeaned. On the other hand, even though the deflecting person seems to be protecting him/herself, he/she does not get the love, appreciation, and tolerance he/she wants in this way and feels lonely. The opposite of deflection, which is "taking in" everything that comes from outside and being affected by everything, can also lead to problems if employed frequently. Since the person cannot decide what is important and what is not, he/she takes the responsibility even though it is not necessary and so feels guilty, ashamed, and sorry (Joyce and Sills 2003, 118).

The items related with deflection on the Gestalt Contact Styles Questionnaire (Revised), which was confirmed as reliable and valid by Aktaş and Daş (2002), are given below. Would you like to mark the items and find out how often you use deflection as a style of contact?

While answering, after reading each point, circle the letter that best reflects your status. The meaning of each letter is as follows:

A: Quite appropriate for me
B: Appropriate for me
C: I am undecided
D: Not appropriate for me
E: Not appropriate for me at all

1.	I have difficulty in completing tasks.	A B C D E
2.	I am late for most things.	A B C D E
3.	It is hard for me to take affairs seriously.	A B C D E
4.	People accuse me of being lazy.	A B C D E
5.	I generally do not know what I really want.	A B C D E
6.	I find it difficult to decide between two opposing views.	A B C D E
7.	I cannot concentrate and cannot focus on an issue.	A B C D E
8.	When faced with a difficult subject, rather than giving up, I generally try to understand it.	A B C D E
9.	I have a tendency to postpone the things I should do.	A B C D E
10.	It is already too late by the time I have thought what to say.	A B C D E
11.	I cannot foresee what the others will say or how they will act.	A B C D E
12.	I find it difficult to understand what I am really feeling.	A B C D E
13.	Sometimes, when the atmosphere becomes stressful, I start laughing.	A B C D E

The scores of the items are A=1, B=2, C=3, D=4, E=5. Only in items 3, 8, and 9 is reverse scoring used. That is, for those items the scoring is thus: A=5, B=4, C=3, D=2 and E=1. The maximum score you can get from these points is 65. The higher your score is, the more you use deflection as a style of contact.

The Basis of Deflection

Deflection as a style of contact can be learned in childhood as well as in other stages of development. However, this style of contact starts to be settled primarily during childhood if the feelings, thoughts, and needs of the child are ignored, not taken into consideration, and when the child is even made to feel guilty and ashamed of them. Under normal conditions, parents are expected to meet the physical, social, mental, and emotional needs of the child, but if such needs are not met, that is, if the child is neglected, then he/she withdraws into his/her own world and starts not to hear the negative reactions coming from outside in order to protect him/herself against these accusing and shaming external reactions. According to Clarkson (1991, 81–82), even if there is not a great deal of criticism and shaming, lack of sufficient positive feedback to the child could lead to his/her frequent use of deflection. Children who get no positive feedback, after a while, become used to not expecting such feedback from the environment, and eventually, even if something positive is said, they start not to believe what they hear. Hence, it is possible to get a totally unexpected reply to a favorable comment from a person who grew up in such an environment. For example, when you say to a friend, "What a nice outfit, it really suits you," he/she, without hearing the compliment, could reply, "You mean this outfit? I just got it from somewhere I don't even remember, it is actually very old," which makes him/herself, you, and your opinions insignificant. Similarly, when you say to someone, "What a good speech!" you may end up with a deflected response such as "Really? Anybody, even the most stupid, can make a speech like this," without any acceptance of the positive feedback. Kepner (1987, 17) indicated that abused children use the deflection mechanism more frequently than most. Children who have experienced emotional, physical, or sexual abuse could choose to react as if they have never experienced or experiencing such abuse in order to deal with the consequent pain and sorrow and not to be affected by them. Similarly, children, though not abused themselves but exposed to physical violence, emotional negligence, or verbal attacks between parents or siblings, deflection can be frequently used.

Personality Characteristics of People Who Use the Deflection Style of Contact Frequently

The deflection style of contact is most clearly observed in the manner of speech of a person. Deflecting people choose roundabout ways, have a tendency to find a thousand excuses in their interactions, and it is really quite difficult to understand what they actually mean. During interaction, they avoid eye contact and prefer to talk in abstract and vague terms. Some of them consider themselves to be well-spoken and humorous talkers. During interpersonal interaction, in order to stay away from a possible intensive contact, they act as if they are very busy, eat something, watch television, and read books or magazines. In these ways, they avoid situations that would expose them to dense and irritating feelings. Kepner (1982) stated that such people are in emotional turmoil, respond with roundabout or vague answers when asked what they are feeling, and in particular avoid focusing on their feelings. In this way, they avoid taking responsibility for their feelings, thoughts, and behaviors. Some people only receive the positive feedback that comes from the outside but do not even hear the negative, while others only receive the negative feedback coming from those who are acting in a jealous or hostile manner and ignore the positive from reliable and warm people. Some others close themselves to any type of criticism coming from the environment and thus do not receive any negative feedback but also become closed to positive reactions such as love and appreciation.

Families that use deflection are often not even aware of problems. In such families, feelings—including care, appreciation, and even anger— are not expressed. The home has a cold and silent atmosphere. Some couples talk about their relationship using statements such as "We never argue" and even present this as a good thing. However, the reason behind not arguing is mostly not "being in agreement" but the avoidance of problems, feelings, and needs through deflection. Some families are too focused on details. In such homes, all the energy is spent on cleaning, tidiness, food, and the like, and thus the main problems are avoided. Some other families, despite their various problems (such as the alcohol problem of the father, passive personality traits of the mother, economic problems, and so on) focus on the outcome of these problems, such as the failure of the child, rather than the prevailing problems. In this way, the child is delegated as the scapegoat and is accused as if his/her failure is the cause of all the family's problems. In some other families, there are sensitive subjects such as deaths, illnesses, money, in-laws, sex, and the like. Talking about these subjects is nearly impossible for such household. Even if the subject comes up, at least one family member continually tries to change the subject, to divert it or cover it up. For example, Patricia, who came to therapy because of depression, told how, except the first year of their six-year married life, they had no intercourse because of the reluctance of her husband and how they had never talked about it over the past five years. When Patricia tried to bring up the subject, however rarely, her husband said, "Stop bothering with these details," and used to leave the room. Sylvia's marriage, on the other hand, was really on the rocks. However, her husband was neither trying to fix the marriage nor asking for any help. When Sylvia wanted to talk about the problems in their relationship, her husband would start to yawn and this yawning would sometimes go on steadily for an hour. Charlotte and Joseph had applied for therapy because of their marital problems. There was a coldness and lack of communication between them. When the reasons for this were being explored, it was revealed that two years previously, they had lost two of their children in a traffic accident and since that day they had never talked about it. Each was unable to broach the subject in order not to make the other one sad and because of their self-blame. As all these examples show, spouses or families who deflect cannot focus on a certain issue and thus cannot solve their problems. In homes where deflection is used frequently as a style of contact, members feel that they cannot reach each other and they are not being heard. It is as if every individual is listening to him/herself, sentences are left incomplete, conversations start in midsentence, the subject is constantly diverted to other areas, or as everybody is talking at the same time, nobody listens to anybody else.

How to Work with Deflection in Therapy

The purpose of work carried out in therapy on deflection is first to make the person aware of the fact that he/she is deflecting, then define the feelings, thoughts, and needs that have led to these deflections, and finally, by facing his/her deflections, to enable the client to take the responsibility of them (Polster and Polster 1974, 90–92). While working with deflection, the therapist has to be an excellent observer and listener and should particularly be highly sensitive to disruptions that might emerge during I-Thou dialogues, as they can provide significant clues about deflections. For example, if a client finds it difficult to continue talking on the same subject and jumps from subject to subject, the therapist should investigate whether or not he/she is avoiding talking about this specific issue, i.e., whether there is deflection. Or, when the therapist asks a question about a certain subject, for example, about the client's family, if the client starts talking about his/her job, the therapist should explore whether or not there is deflection. It can be discovered not only through verbal clues but also by observation of body language. For example, the client's avoidance of eye contact with the therapist during the session may be deflection. When the therapist becomes aware of the fact that the client is avoiding eye contact, then he/she can share this observation with the client if it is seen as significant. In some other situations, the client could be deflecting with distracting body movements such as twiddling one's thumbs or swinging the legs. In such cases, the therapist can share these observations to help the client to be aware of his/her deflection. While working with deflecting clients, the therapist should also be a model to the client by not allowing the subject to be digressed from and the contact to be disrupted.

Once the client becomes aware of his/her deflections, then it is time to work on their meaning (Crocker 1999, 101). Now the emphasis is on from what the client is trying to protect him/herself or to avoid. For example, when the client in the above example was asked, "I asked you a question about your family and you started talking about your job. Does this mean anything to you?" the answer was, "then I would have to put down my family and I would never want to do it." Again, when a client avoiding eye contact was asked, "I am aware that you are not looking at me, is there something which prevents you from doing that?" the client's reply was, "Then you would have seen that I was about to cry and I would have been very ashamed of this." Some people could be deflecting because they think that they can protect their relationship by avoiding arguments, and some do so to avoid feeling guilty after an argument. Some others deflect because they assume that they will make the other person unhappy if they express their feelings. Again some others choose this route because they really do not know what to do or to say. However, whatever the reason, it is clear that deflection protects the person against rejection, exclusion, abandonment, or negative feelings in general.

At the next stage, work is carried out on these negative feelings that the person is avoiding. In the Gestalt approach, it is believed that instead of avoiding feelings, it is necessary to accept them, to experience them, and thus to "consume" them. Hence, in therapy, facing out the negative feelings is especially important in order to help the client to articulate and experience them. To this end, for example, with the client who said he/she would have put down his/her family, work is carried out on why he/she would have to demean the family and what this means to him/her on one hand, while on the other hand, work is carried out on the feelings that have emerged during this work. While working with deflections, very often unfinished business emerges. For example, the client mentioned above, while answering the question as to why he would have put down his parents explained in tears how, as a child, he frequently had to witness arguments between his parents that included physical violence. In such cases, it is possible to make use of empty chair and imagination experiments in order to complete the unfinished business of the person with his parents, by having him express his previously held-back feelings and thoughts. Sometimes, the client could be asked to remember a conversation where he/she deflected and then wanted to discuss that subject in a different manner this time without deflecting by using the two-chair method. The two chair method can also be carried out in a case where not the client but the other person is deflecting to create a new way to communicate with the other person. And in couple therapy, the couple can be invited to discuss a subject that so far they have been unable to talk about because they deflect. Work carried out with the above-mentioned Charlotte and Joseph who lost two children in a traffic accident can be given as an example here. In therapy, when the couple was asked to share their feelings about the accident, they could not start talking for a long time (about ten minutes). Both were looking down, playing with their hands, and were absolutely silent. Through the whole session, both of them were in tears. Joseph was the first to start talking:

Joseph: *I am very sorry. I don't know what to say. I am sorry.*

Charlotte: (after a four-minute silence) *I am also very sorry. I miss them so much.*

Joseph: *I miss them very much too. Even looking at their pictures burns me inside. I just burn* (silence). *I wish I was the one who had died instead of them.*

Charlotte: (in a very low voice) *I wish that too. This is God's punishment for me. I didn't die and I am living with this. If we didn't have our third daughter, if we didn't have Jane . . . I considered dying so many times, but . . .*

Joseph: *Remember I came home very late that day, at seven in the morning. I walked the streets the whole night. I went to the site of the accident. I wanted to jump in front of a car and to be run down. I rebelled against God. I begged him to take my life also. I couldn't tell you when I came home. You were not talking either. You were sitting with Jane on your lap. I was even angry with Jane. If she hadn't been there, death would have been so easy for me. Then I was ashamed of being angry with Jane. I couldn't look at either of your faces. I couldn't face anybody.*

Charlotte: *I keep blaming myself. If only I had been more careful. I wish we hadn't taken that street. I wouldn't have bought those ice creams.*

Joseph: *I am the one to blame. I should have been taking you to school that day. I wish I hadn't had that errand to run. I am the one who is guilty, how can you take three kids to school by yourself. I should have taken care of you all.*

Charlotte: (looks at her husband for the first time) *What nonsense. I am a grown up woman. I should have taken care of them. You weren't even there.*

Joseph: *I should have been. I should have. You must be very angry with me for this. You would be right never to forgive me*

Charlotte: *Why should I be angry with you? I am angry with myself. Actually you are the one who would be right if you never forgive me. I don't forgive myself anyway.*

(At this point, I reminded them that the accident happened because the brakes of the minibus that hit the children failed.)

Joseph: *Even if this is true, it is still my fault.*
If I were a more resourceful man, than.....

Charlotte: *You are actually. Don't be ridiculous. Remember how you made a doll's buggy for Judith* [their oldest daughter]. *Then Kate* [their second daughter] *also played with it. Even Jane was playing with it until I got fed up and threw it away.*

Joseph: *I wish they were alive and I would make another one. I made it, so what?* (Looks at his wife for the first time)

Charlotte: *I just can't take this pain. I can't even go to their graves. I want to go so much, but I just can't. We never went.*

Joseph: *I did, I go. On their birthdays, on anniversaries of their deaths, I didn't tell you so as not to make you sad, but I went many times to the cemetery.*

Charlotte: (after a long silence) *Take me also, let us go. They are our children. They live inside me, but they are there. Take me too, please?*

They were now looking at each other and holding hands while talking. At the end of the session, they set a date for the cemetery visit and planned a new doll's buggy for Jane to be made by Joseph. This was a session where very intense feelings were shared. By the time of their next appointment, they had visited the cemetery and Joseph had made the buggy. They continued to share their feelings about the loss of their children in the following session.

While working with deflection, another point that should be considered is to make the person aware of what he/she is missing while trying to protect him/herself through deflection. For this purpose, for example while working with Patricia, who had had no sex with her husband for five years, the first work was on what she gained by not talking about the issue and by not having sex. Patricia stated that by not talking about this issue, she was protecting her marriage because she did not want to be a divorced woman, and also she did not know how she could explain the situation to her parents and did not want to worry them. She added that, as they were known as a very happy couple, she did not want to change this image of theirs. On the other hand, she realized that by not talking and forcing the issue, she was losing her chance of having a baby, her femininity, her self-confidence, her spontaneity and joy. In some cases, after a person becomes aware of what he/she is protecting and what is being missed, he/she might remain in an impasse for a while. How to work with impasses in therapy will be given in the section on resistance.

By working on deflection in therapy, the deflected energy is directed to the correct target, and thus contact is achieved. From there on, the person starts not to feel the need for deflection as a means of protection, to express him/herself in more active ways, to focus on his/her problems, and to be willing to resolve conflicts in a mutually satisfactory manner. This means that after work carried out on deflection, the person learns not to be afraid of negative feelings and feedback and how to enjoy positive feedback.

11

PROJECTION

What Is Projection?

In its most general sense, projection is the process of interpreting people, objects, and incidents in the environment depending on one's own knowledge and experiences. Projection, or the process of interpretation, can occur in various ways:

   a.   Speculating about the future or planning is a form of projection. For example, before going on a trip, we pack our bags according to our speculations about what we are going to do at the destination, what the weather will be like, the characteristics of the place to be visited, etc. When we want to surprise a friend or when we are getting a gift for someone, we guess what that person would like, that is, we project our knowledge about that person into the future and make our choice accordingly. Again, when playing chess, when we think, "If I make this move, then he will respond with such a move and I can beat him," then what we are doing is projection. Fortune-telling is also another type of projection.

   b.   Artistic endeavors such as painting, sculpting, the writing of poetry, stories or novels, or dancing are also examples of projection. For example, a painter projects his/her feelings and thoughts into the picture being created. An architect, while designing a building, in addition to his/her professional knowledge, also projects the features he/she considers beautiful and significant into the design.

c. Guessing what another person is thinking, feeling, or why he/she is acting in a certain manner is also projection. For example, at a gathering, when you see someone approaching you with a smile and an extended hand, based on your past experiences, you might think that he/she is well-meaning and acting in a friendly way, thus, when you extend your hand with a smile, you are projecting. To come to the conclusion that your child loves documentaries after he/she has been watching a documentary about animals for a long time is also a form of projection.

d. Your comments about people you do not know well, subjects you have no idea or incidents you have not witnessed are again projections. For example when you think how loving or haughty someone you have just met is or when you are commenting on the economy of your country even though you are not an economist or when you are gossiping, this is again projection.

e. Prejudices or extreme generalizations are other examples of projection. For example, to be a fanatical fan of a certain football team, to put down those who are not of your religious persuasion, to demean those who are from a certain race or sex, and to judge those who dress in a certain way are all projections. Here the person is attributing those aspects of him/herself that he/she disowns to another group, opinion, or belief. Similarly to sublimate and to overappreciate those who are similar, who feel and act in the same way is also projecting.

f. Most of the accusations we direct at others are also projection. For example when we say to somebody, "You are so selfish,", we are accusing him/her of not being considerate to us, but this actually shows that we are also selfish because, with this accusation, we are saying, "Don't think about yourself, think about me," which is an act of projecting our own selfishness onto the other person. Jealousy among spouses is also projection-based. In such cases, instead of reviewing and strengthening our self-confidence, we project our insecurity onto our partner by accusation. In other words, since we do not like ourselves, we think that our partners will also not like us or will like other men or women more. Sometimes the reason behind our accusing somebody is the fact that they are able to behave in ways we do not allow ourselves to behave. For example, when a friend is late, without even asking why he/she was late, we may accuse him/her of not being prompt and may even portray ourselves as righteous by saying, "I am never late to a meeting." In truth, everybody can be late to a meeting from time to time and this is not the end of the world. However, if we believe that being late is a very bad thing, by always avoiding it—that is, by never doing something "bad"—we feel "good," and while feeling good, we do not care if the other person is feeling bad. That is to say, with the expectation of being "punished" by others if we are late, we are never late and by projecting this expectation onto others, we "punish" them.

g. Loading the responsibility of our feelings and actions onto others is also projection. For example with remarks such as, "Don't make me mad," "You've made my blood pressure go up," or "Don't mess with my mind," we submit the control of our temper, blood pressure and mind to others, and thus we project our vulnerability and weakness onto them.

h. While we can project our characteristics, feelings, thoughts, and beliefs onto other people and objects, we can also project them onto our bodies. For example, when we say, "My heart is heavy," "My head aches," or "My body is tired," we have projected the heaviness, ache or tiredness to various parts of our body.

As can be understood from the above examples, projection is a style of contact used very often in daily life. According to Polster and Polster (1974, 82), "each person is in the center of gravity of his/her universe, and creates his/her world where he/she is the center of gravity." Korb et al. (1989, 57) have also stated that people create their own world through projections that are depending on their perceptions, beliefs, attitudes, feelings and images. Kepner (1982) claims that a continuously projecting person is as if living in a house full of mirrors and, every time he/she looks in a mirror thinks that he/she is not seeing him/herself but somebody else. According to Naranjo (1995: 142) projections are at the same time a reality and an illusion. They are real because the person cannot project something he/she does not know or has not experienced onto somebody else or to an object or a situation, and in that sense, projections are images of inner experiences. They are illusions because the characteristics attributed to another person, object, or situation generally do not belong to that person, object, or situation. In conclusion, moving on from all this information, we can say that a person determines his/her life and relations according to his/her projections.

The Advantages and Disadvantages of Projection

Projections can both facilitate and complicate a person's life and relations. If the projections enable the person to make realistic plans, to better organize his/her future, to establish more satisfactory relationships with those around him/herself, to meet his/her needs, to be creative and productive, then they are advantageous; otherwise they are disadvantageous. Korb et al. (1989, 57) group the projections as healthy or unhealthy, accurate or distorted, and functional or nonfunctional. In cases of unhealthy, distorted, or nonfunctional projections, the person attributes the characteristics, attitudes, feelings, or behaviors that he/she posses but refuses to acknowledge to the people or objects around. Thus, the person behaving as if these projections have nothing to do with him/her feels relieved (Perls et al. 1951/1996, 221). In other words the projecting person

- is aware of his or her characteristics, attitudes, feelings, and behaviors,
- does not want to acknowledge their existence as he or she dislikes them,
- consequently, expresses them as if they belong to somebody else.

It is so much easier for a projecting person to think that "badness" lies with someone else rather than accepting that he or she is "bad."

Fighting with somebody else needs much less energy than fighting with one's self. Furthermore, fighting with the self is a lonely process and causes anxiety, while accusing another person is much more comforting (Zinker 1977, 206)

In terms of Gestalt therapy, as these types of projections are harmful as they prevent the integration of personality and the person- environment contact in particular (Sills et al. 1998, 63). Those who establish contact through projection, instead of contacting other people by exploring their feelings, thoughts, and behaviors, form an "imaginary" relationship according to their own perceptions. In this relationship, they take the characteristics that they neither like nor accept as the basis of contact. Perls (1969a/1992) indicated that people who use a projection style of contact frequently turn the world into a war zone. For example, the person who thinks that others envy him/her is actually refusing to accept that he/she is the one who is envying them; someone who says, "My father does not show his love, he doesn't love me," is actually refusing to accept that he/she is the one who does not show his/her love to his/her father and does not love him; the woman who claims that "men regard women as very weak" is actually refusing to accept that she is the one who finds women weak. Again, a person who thinks crying is a weakness and who demeans those who cry is actually the one who wants to cry but, due to his/her various fears, does not permit him/herself to cry and projects his/her anger onto those who cry; or a person who feels anger toward those who are overweight is actually the one who wants to eat a lot but, again due to a multitude of fears, does not allow him/herself to eat as much as he/she wants and therefore demeans those who eat as they please.

People not only project the negative characteristics that they cannot accept but may also project the positive traits that they cannot integrate within their personality onto others (Sills et al. 1998, 63). For example, a man who is actually very good-looking can be jealous of a "handsome" man around him since he does not believe that he is good-looking and by finding another excuse—such as claiming that the other is very cocky— can turn his anger toward him. Similarly, a person who refuses to believe that he/she is smart, even though he/she has always got good grades and successfully graduated from several schools, can believe that everybody thinks that he/she is stupid.

In short, the projecting person denies his/her anger, defensiveness, sexuality, love, compassion, or any other characteristic and attributes them to someone else. A healthy person, whether they are acceptable or not, is aware of his/her feelings, thoughts, beliefs, and needs and tests whether he/she is projecting these onto another person, object, or situation in a correct way. In other words, the healthy position is to observe what "really" happens, to recognize these observations, to be aware of the projections, to take the responsibility of them, and to be open to new information (Korb et al. 1989, 58). The person who contacts through projection assumes and is even sure that he or she genuinely knows what others feel, what they think, and why they behave as they do and that he or she can read others' minds. This causes him/her to develop an inflated self and an exaggerated personality. If this becomes chronic or severe, then it can lead to paranoia or psychotic delusions (Kepner 1982). In such cases, the person generally believes that others will do something harmful to him/her. However, the person's belief that others will do him/her harm actually indicates that he/she wants to do harmful things to others (Perls 1973, 35).

The Basis of Projection

Introjections are at the base of projections (Perls 1973, 35). The strong influence of parents on children during childhood was discussed in the section on introjections. What we introject is determined by the reactions shown to us by our parents and others who are important in our lives, and consequently when we grow up, we think that those around us will behave in the same way (Sills et al. 1968, 63). For example, when a client who cries during therapy says to the therapist, "Because I complain so much, you must be thinking of me as a very weak person," he/she is projecting the introjected message of "people who complain are weak" that he/she learned from his/her father in his/her childhood to the therapist. At this point, the client almost sees his father's face superimposed on that of the therapist. In such a situation, if the therapist says, "I don't think that you are weak at all because you complain" the client might be quite surprised and might not even believe what the therapist is saying since the projecting people are so sure of the thoughts they are projecting that they do not bother to investigate whether or not they are correct.

According to Polster and Polster (1974, 78), there are many "shoulds" and "shouldn'ts" at the base of projections. "I should not express my anger," "Men should not show their feelings," and "Women should be ladylike" can be given as examples of this. A person who believes that he/she should not express anger will obviously refrain from showing it to others and may even try not to feel angry; by projecting this feeling onto other person will think that it is the other who is angry with him/her. A man, who believes that men should not show their feelings, will be irritated by those who can articulate their emotions and may even accuse them of being "womanly." A woman who believes that women should be ladylike will refuse to acknowledge those feelings and desires (for example, her sexual desires) that do not fit her definition of "ladylike" and, by projecting them onto men, will claim that all men are sex fiends. The person whose identity is occupied with such information deceives him/herself for life through the projections he/she makes. Since the person attributes the feelings and impulses he/she possesses but refuses to accept onto others by projection, thinks that he/she has the right to criticize others and sees him/herself as superior.

Personality Characteristics of People Who Use the Projection Style of Contact Frequently

The most distinctive characteristic of people who use the projection style of contact frequently is the accusing of other people and the environment in many areas. Since such people believe that problems are always caused by others and that they are "innocent," they think that the solutions should also be found by others. Hence they see themselves as victims of circumstances and other people and thus cannot actively participate in life (Perls 1973, 35). In other words, those who use projection frequently believe that control of their lives is not in their own hands but lies with other people or things and hence by avoiding responsibility they put themselves in a passive position (Perls et al. 1951/1996, 211). They generally use sentences that are not in the first person but the second or third, such as, "You don't understand me,"

"You are treating me badly," "He wants to use me," or "They reject me." Although accusing others and not taking responsibility make the person feel fine, this causes at the same time feelings of weakness and helplessness. Clarkson and Mackewn (1993, 74) stated that those who frequently use projection are oversuspicious, cautious, prejudiced, and tense people who constantly complain.

McConville (1995, 150) stated that, in families where members use projection frequently, everybody is focused on the problems of others, and hence, the family members are not aware of their inner experiences and problems. In such families, when a problem arises, everybody accuses everybody else and nobody shows an effort to actually resolve the problem. Each person expects somebody else to do this, and nobody wants to see his/her part in the roots of the problem. In some families that frequently use this style of contact, one of the members is chosen as the scapegoat and that person is seen as the cause of all the problems arising in the family. On the other hand, the member chosen as the scapegoat continually accuses the others in turn. In these families where a hostile attitude prevails, nobody takes responsibility.

How to Work with Projection in Therapy

According to the Gestalt therapy approach, everybody should take responsibility for his/her life, feelings, thoughts, and behavior. We can find the courage to change the world we have created only if we can take on this responsibility (Polster and Polster 1974, 78). By refraining from taking responsibility for the feelings, thoughts, and behaviors that they possess but do not approve of and by not believing that they can change their lives, people who project attribute those parts of themselves that they don't like or want, to others. However, it is not possible to get rid of them by refusing to acknowledge their existence or by attributing them to others. The only way to get rid of the unwanted parts is to accept them, to express them, and to integrate them in the personality (Perls et al. 1951/1996, 221). Hence the goal targeted during therapy related to projection is to help the client to become aware of these rejected parts, to express them, and to integrate them within him/herself.

It is obvious that is not worked on all the projections of the client in therapy since there are a lot of projections that is used in daily life and some of them make the life easier. However, if the projections are obstructing the person's contact with others and preventing him/her from having satisfactory relationships, then it is necessary to work on them. Recognizing projections is not at all easy because, through them, people protect and justify themselves. Furthermore, there might be a realistic aspect of the projections. For example, when we say, "He is treating me badly," that person could really be doing so, but this does not change the fact that we may also treating him badly. We can sometimes say, "If he does not treat me badly, then I will not treat him badly," but this does not mean other than our putting the responsibility for our bad treatment onto the other person; furthermore, it does not take us to a solution. In therapy, in order to help clients to be aware of their projections, first of all, a very good therapist-client relationship must be established and the client has to be sure of the therapist's support (Perls et al. 1951/1996, 214). The purpose of projection work is not to have the person feel guilty or to accuse him/herself, but quite the contrary, to learn to be tolerant of him/herself. In the Gestalt approach, there is no room for interpretations because they are themselves the projections of the person who is doing the interpreting. Hence, the therapist should also be aware of his/her projections and should have integrated them into his/her personality.

Various experiments can be used during therapy to enable the client to recognize and articulate his/her projections. One of them is related to the language used. As mentioned above, projecting people have a tendency to use pronouns other than "I" and to attribute responsibility to other people or situations. Consequently one of the purposes of language experiments is to help the person to take responsibility by using the first person pronoun. To that end, for example, when the client says, "He does not understand me," the therapist could ask the client to change it into "I don't understand him." Similarly, the therapist could ask the client to rephrase the statement "My parents want me to be very successful" into "I want myself to be very successful," "an annoying situation" into "I am annoyed by this situation," or "Society does not approve this behavior" into "I don't approve this behavior." During therapy, another area where language experiments are used is projections onto the body. Here the purpose is to integrate "I" and the body, or in other words, the body and the mind (Kepner 1987, 113). For example, the therapist could ask the client to say, "I am giving myself a headache" when he/she says "I have a headache," or to say, "I am tightening my throat," when he/she says,

"My throat is tight." Later, the client might be asked to complete these expressions in different forms or to further clarify them, as in, "I am giving myself a headache because I don't trust you" or "I am tightening my throat so that I can prevent myself from expressing my anger to you."

One other method that can be used in enabling the client to become aware of his/her projections is the empty chair technique. During this experiment, the client imagines that the person with whom he/she particularly feels helpless, sad, angry, or rejected is sitting in the empty chair and he/she starts to explain his/her feelings as well as what he/she wants to say. In some cases, two chair technique can also be used. In this experiment after the client expressed what he/she wanted to express to the other person in the empty chair, then he or she takes the other person's place and talking and behaving as that person answers him/herself. Through these experiments, the client starts to own some of the characteristics of the person he/she was projecting onto or rather his/her own characteristics that were being projected. As an example, part of the session with Mike, who is generally very quiet and unaware of his anger, is given below. At the beginning of the session, Mike mentioned that he had gone to see his father who had treated him very angrily. Upon this, he was asked to imagine that his father was sitting in the empty chair and then to move to that chair and to repeat in the same tone of voice, with the same facial expression and manner, what his father had said to him that day and to establish a dialogue between himself and his father.

Mike (as his father): (speaking loudly) *Where have you been? I hardly see you. How can a son never call his father? You won't know if I'm dead or alive.*

Mike (as himself): (speaking in a low voice) *What can I do, Father? I didn't have time. I have so much work; I can't keep up with it.*

Mike (as his father): (speaking even more loudly) *What rubbish! Everybody is very busy. I have a lot of work to do. You are a scapegrace, that is why. You don't care about anybody but yourself.*

Mike (as himself):	(in a low voice and looking down*) All right, Father. But I was very busy. You are busy too, of course.*
Mike (as his father):	(with an angry expression) *No, no. This is just an excuse, an excuse for not seeing me. You are only thinking of yourself—you are selfish.*
Mike (as himself):	(speaking loudly) *Actually it is you who does not care about anybody but yourself. There are such good fathers. You could also have called me, but you wouldn't do that. Why?* (his voice became louder, his face started to flush, and he started to breathe more rapidly) *Would the telephone stick to your hand, or is it too expensive? But you spend money on other things like going out, taking others out for a meal. You have both money and time for that, don't you?*
Mike (as his father):	*As if you are any different. You went on a vacation just last week. What was it? Just a weekend trip! Did you even once ask me to go on a vacation with you?*

During this dialogue, Mike realized that neither he nor his father was very willing to call the other and also how they were accusing each other by projecting their own reluctance to call. Another point Mike became aware of was the fact that not only was his father very angry with him but that the opposite was also the case—he had a lot of anger toward his father. Although Mike never raised his voice to his father in his daily life, while talking as his father during this dialogue, he found out that he could talk more loudly if he wanted and how he could show his anger to his father. Later, the dialogue continued as follows:

Mike (as himself):	*I will not call you as long as you don't call me. You are the father; you are the one who should call.*

Mike (as his father):	*Well, you are twenty-eight years old. You are a grown man. You are not a child! But you call when you have a problem. Do I interfere with your life? I am not asking whether or not you went out to dinner, with whom you went, how much you paid. I just listen if you tell me.*
Mike (as himself):	*Of course you don't ask. You don't have the time to ask. You do not ask because you are afraid that I might ask for something.*
Mike (as his father):	*Did I ever refuse an invitation from you? Did I ever refuse to do something that you asked for? I took your car to be fixed just the other day.*
Mike (as himself):	*So what? You were the one who knew the mechanic. He works faster and for less money because you know him. Now you fling it in my teeth. Well, he didn't do a good job with the car anyway.*
Mike (as his father):	*And that is my fault too! He is a good mechanic. I don't know what he failed to fix, but you should have said something.*
Mike (as himself):	*Why should I tell him? You should have told him, he is your man.*

During this dialogue, Mike became aware of the role he was playing in the occurrence of the negative communication between his father and himself and how much he was expecting from his father. Realizing this helped him to come out of the "helpless victim" role and to develop active strategies about how he should act in his relationship with his father. That is, projection was replaced with coping.

Art work is another method that can be used in therapy to raise awareness of projections. One of the most widely used art practices during therapy is asking the client to draw. The therapist could ask the client to draw anything he or she wants to or could be more guiding and ask the client for a picture of a tree, an animal they like, his/her feelings, impasse, or resistance. In some cases, depending on what the client needs, he/she might be asked to draw someone he/she does not like or an incident that made him/her unhappy. At the base of all art work lies the point of view that the person is projecting something from his or her inner world into the picture he/she draws. Later, while working on these drawings, what the client has reflected about him/herself in these pictures is explored and thus, increasing the client's awareness about him/herself is targeted.

Another method that can be utilized during therapy is to make the client act, talk, or behave like the person he/she particularly dislikes in order to help the client to be aware of what he/she has projected onto this person, or in other words to be aware of which traits or characteristics he/she does not accept. For this purpose, for example, the client might be asked to behave like the boss he/she cannot stand. This practice could be initially hard for the clients, but it is very helpful in terms of raising the clients' awareness of what they project onto others and then integrating those characteristics by acknowledging them. In the acknowledgment of projections and their integration within the personality, group work is also very effective. According to the Gestalt approach, projections also form the basis of dreams, and these can be worked in various ways during therapy either individually or in groups. How this can be done is discussed in detail in the section on dreams.

In conclusion, acceptance of projections will help the person to have a more flexible and enriched personality. Thus, by becoming aware of the traits that were previously unacknowledged because he or she did not like them and that were remain in the dark, the client will be able to come out of the "helpless victim" role, and by integrating these traits within his/her personality, he or she will become a more powerful person who can accept him/herself as he or she is and who can take his/her own responsibilities in life. Integrating the projected parts within the personality brings freedom of choice to the person.

12

RETROFLECTION

What Is Retroflection?

Under normal conditions, when a need becomes apparent, energy is released, and the person is mobilized to meet this need. However, in the style of contact known as retroflection, instead of orienting the energy to be used for his or her needs to the environment, the person directs it at him/herself. Individuals who direct their energy at themselves cut off their contact with the environment and, by focusing on their own feelings and thoughts, withdraw and become immobilized (Sills et al. 1998, 65). The most important outcome of retroflection is the prevention of the person's ability to mobilize to meet his or her needs (Clarkson 1991, 54). Although many people are aware of their needs they lack the strength to mobilize themselves to meet them. For example, expressions such as "I want to attend a guitar course but can never find the time," "I know it is time to break up with him, but I can't help myself from talking as if nothing is wrong when he calls" or "These days I just don't want to do anything, I can't even study" can be frequently heard. Behind all these expressions actually lies the complaint "I want to but I can't." People who use this type of expression are blocking their energy instead of using it to satisfy their needs (Kepner 1987, 149).

There are two types of retroflection (Polster and Polster 1974, 86). In the first case, as the person is unable to direct his or her energy to the main target, or believes that this would not be appropriate, he or she directs this energy to him/herself. That is, he or she tells or does to him/herself what he or she actually wants to say or do to others. For example, let us assume that you are very hurt because of something done by someone you love. In such a situation, what needs to be done is to talk to the loved one about the issue in question, tell that person your feelings, find out why he or she behaved in that way, and try to understand each other because you need each other's attention and love. However, in such a situation if you deny your need for his/her love and attention and instead of expending your energy on talking to him or her, if you hold it inside and feel offended, then you will be directing your energy at yourself. Similarly, when you face any failure, instead of mobilizing to find out the causes of this failure, if you expend your energy on thoughts such as "I am stupid anyway, I can't succeed in anything," you are again retroflecting.

In the second type of retroflection, people treat their environment as they themselves want to be treated. For example, some people never criticize others as they hate to be criticized, or they never argue with anybody because facing another's anger bothers them greatly. Again, some others are always attentive to others because they themselves need attention.

There are also situations where both types of retroflection are used simultaneously. For example, in order to get attention, Ellen was always helping those around her and dealing with their problems. In return, when people were attentive to her, she would start to blame herself, thinking, "Am I being selfish?" or "Do I deserve this attention?" As she was actually blaming others without even being aware of it for not being attentive to her unless she was to them, and as she could not express these unnoticed feelings, she was turning the blame on herself. It is clear that in both cases, Ellen was unable to meet her need for attention in a satisfactory way.

When a person becomes aware of a certain need, his or her failure to eagerly mobilize to satisfy that need is due to an underlying feeling of anxiety. Beneath this feeling of anxiety, on the other hand, lies the inadequacy of the existing self-support systems of the person, in addition to negative beliefs regarding his or her capacity to cope with possible future situations; or in other words, the person's introjections (Perls et al. 1951/1996, 129). The causes of the repression of feelings and the inability to express them are catastrophic expectations, i.e., pertaining to negative possibilities and the fear that accompanies them. In those who frequently use a retroflective style of contact, the reason for their inability to express feelings, thoughts, and desires to those around them with the aim of meeting their needs and of their failure to mobilize is their various anxieties, fears, and catastrophic expectations. When regarded from a social perspective, the needs, thoughts, and desires that are hardest to express are those related to anger and sex. Self-righteousness, self-worth, assertiveness, tenderness, and love are also difficult to express (Zinker 1977, 102). Many people believe that if they voice their anger, they will harm or destroy the world around them; if they express their sexuality, they will be seen as manic or perverted; if they express their love, they will bore and suffocate others; if they indulge in self-praise, they will be either excluded or teased. Hence, retroflective people, by not expressing their feelings and desires, do not use their energy outward but rather turn it inward. In truth, there is no problem in expressing needs and desires to others at an appropriate time and in an appropriate manner, and this is actually the only way to satisfy these needs. According to the Gestalt approach, in order to grow and integrate, the person has to be in contact with his/her environment and has to direct his/her energy outward.

In retroflection, the person's energy is trapped between two opposing forces (Kepner 1993, 150). While one side is saying "do," the other says "don't." Hence the person is stuck between do/don't, stop/act, and yes/no. While on one hand, the person wants to behave in a certain way, such as expressing a feeling or voicing a thought, on the other hand, he/she also expects negative reactions from those around. Hence the person can risk neither giving up these wishes nor actualizing them, and thus the energy that cannot be released is retroflected.

The Advantages and Disadvantages of Retroflection

Retroflection, just like other styles of contact, can be used in either an advantageous or a disadvantageous way for the person. For example, thinking is a form of retroflection (Polster and Polster 1974, 85). Retroflection is involved even in thoughts that lead to very simple decisions such as "Which TV channel should I watch this evening?" While thinking can have adverse effects such as obstructing or postponing mobilization, it can also have a beneficial impact, such as when providing answers to questions which the person has to answer but which are very hard to resolve on the instant. Self-love, self-admiration, self-approval, and saying nice things to oneself, as well as self-criticism, self-deprecation, suicide, the inability to say "no," self- mutilation, and all types of addictions are examples of retroflection. Whether retroflection is advantageous or disadvantageous for the person depends on the conditions. If retroflection helps the person to increase his or her self-confidence, to be free, to protect him/herself and his/her own boundaries, or to increase his/her skills and talent, then it is beneficial. For example, retroflection is helpful when dieting, for a mother clenching her hands to refrain from spanking her child, or for a staff member holding his/ her tongue to refrain from swearing like a trooper at the boss. If a person consciously chooses to retroflect in a certain situation and if he or she has a rational reason for this, then it is healthy. However, if retroflection has become a habit, became chronic, or used without awareness, then it is harmful and unhealthy. Retroflecting continuously and under all circumstances, i.e., to hold feelings and thoughts within the self, is a stressful situation and eventually leads to psychological problems (Perls et al. 1951/1996, 146). Frequent use of retroflection as a contact style can also cause psychosomatic illnesses, that is to say, physical illnesses with psychological causes (Perls et al. 1951/1996, 162).

The items related with retroflection on the Gestalt Contact Styles Questionnaire (Revised), which was confirmed as reliable and valid by Aktaş and Daş (2002), are given below. Would you like to mark the items and find out how often you use retroflection? While answering, after reading each item, circle the letter that best reflects your status. The meaning of each letter is as follows:

A: Highly appropriate for me
B: Appropriate for me
C: I am undecided
D: Not appropriate for me
E: Not appropriate for me at all

1. I feel rather distant from life and people. A B C D E
2. I frequently realize that I have a problem. A B C D E
3. I feel that I am a victim of circumstances. A B C D E
4. I generally feel guilty or angry. A B C D E
5. I am never satisfied with what I do. A B C D E
6. I think a lot about everything. A B C D E
7. I find it difficult to get rid of those feelings that bother me. A B C D E
8. There are a lot of things I want to do, but I just cannot act. A B C D E
9. I feel dull (stagnant, numb). A B C D E
10. If people really got to know me, they would tell what a tense person I am. A B C D E
11. I get along well with almost everybody. A B C D E
12. People say they find it difficult to understand my point of view. A B C D E
13. I live according to my family's expectations. A B C D E
14. I am not a relaxed person. A B C D E
15. Even when I don't do anything strenuous, my muscles generally hurt. A B C D E
16. I suffer from nausea and stomach pains. A B C D E
17. I wait for others to start conservation. A B C D E
18. The sources of most of my problems are other people. A B C D E

The scores of the points are A=1, B=2, C=3, D=4, E=5. Only in the last item there is a reverse scoring; that is, for this item, the scoring is thus: A=5, B=4, C=3, D=2 and E=1. The maximum score you can get from these items is 90. The higher your score is, the more you use retroflection as a style of contact.

The Basis of Retroflection

Retroflection, as a style of contact, starts to be established with the punishment of the expression of needs during childhood and by the failure and consequent disappointments following repeated attempts of expressing the needs by the child (Perls et al. 1951/1996, 147). Under normal conditions, it is expected that parents take into consideration and meet, as far as possible, the needs and desires of the child. However, the child whose needs and desires are repeatedly unmet for whatever reasons finally learns, not perhaps to forget about his or her needs and desires, but not to express them and instead to hold them back. This is very important particularly in terms of the expression of feelings. For example, when the child's request to sit on his or her mother's or father's lap or to play with them is refused, first he/she becomes insistent. If the child's insistence is dealt with by the parents in a reasonable way, and if the child's distress and anger arising from these refusals is accepted and an effort is made to calm the child down, then there will be no problem. On the other hand, when the child keeps insisting, if the parents' responses are along the lines of "You are asking for too much," or "We are fed up with your demands"; or when the child is crying, if the responses of the parents are "Boys don't cry," "You are such a sissy," or even "If you cry, I will spank you"; that is, if the child is made to feel embarrassed, guilty, or scared and—if the worst comes to the worst— faces abuse, then this child can do nothing but retroflect by holding his/her breath, stopping his/her tears, and keeping his/her anger inside. Polster and Polster (1974, 149) mention that, in such cases, there are two types of retroflection that a child can choose. A child whose feelings, thoughts, and desires are not sufficiently considered and who has met with indifferent and insensitive attitudes can start to think, "Nobody cares for me." If a child thinking along these lines develops a belief that the reason for his/her not being cared for by his/her parents is his/her being "unimportant," then he/she will start to judge, demean, and fail to care about him/herself and to see him/herself as guilty of everything. This is the first retroflection type.

Another child brought up under the same conditions may also get the impression that "nobody cares for me" but, in contrast to the former, reacts with "Then I have to care for myself" and starts to give too much importance and value to him/herself, resulting in self-aggrandizement. However, in this case too, the basic belief, or in Gestalt terminology, the "introjected" message is that "Nobody cares for me"; this child might show narcissistic characteristics and may turn into an "all by myself" person who does not ask for help from anybody. This is the second type of retroflection. Some children brought up under the same conditions and who have the same belief could employ these two types of retroflection simultaneously.

Obstruction of the child's desires and needs, along with the threat of punishment or not being loved, causes the child's energy to be split into two. While part of this energy is used to satisfy the unmet need, the rest goes to keep the need under control. Consequently the initial conflict between the child and the parent in terms of meeting the needs turns in time into a conflict between the part of the child that wants to do and that wants to hold (Perls et al. 1951/1996, 146). Later, even if the child grows, his/her parents will now be far away, and there will be no-one obstructing him/her, he/she keeps on obstructing him/herself because of these inner conflicts; thus, the retroflection style of contact becomes ingrained.

Personality Characteristics of People Who Use the Retroflection Style of Contact Frequently

According to Kepner (1982), those who use the retroflection style of contact frequently blame themselves for many things, even for problems arising from the environment. These individuals are extremely sensitive in terms of their mistakes, faults, or wrongs. Furthermore, the feeling of self-pity is very intense in those who often use the retroflection style of contact. They always make plans and think a lot about the consequences of their behaviors. They are very keen on being in control and very scared of losing or submitting their control, and hence, they are reluctant to take risks. It might be very difficult for these people to ask for something, even if that is attention and love from others. Even though they might seem to be very free, they are actually lonely because establishing contact with other people is very scary for them.

McConville (1995, 156–159) has pointed out that the families where the members frequently use the retroflection style of contact generally pursue a life that is quiet, isolated, closed, and introvert. In these families, the members do not express their feelings and prefer not to talk in order to avoid conflicts. They do not show any empathy for each other, and when a problem arises, they cannot give emotional support to one other. In such families, it is generally expected that every member should deal with the problems on his or her own and never lose control.

Physical Characteristics of People Who Use the Retroflection Style of Contact Frequently

If a person is punished, criticized, or rejected when expressing feelings such as anger, sadness, love, desire, or fear, then that person consequently also tries to stop the expression of these feelings with his/her body (Kepner 1987, 149). For example, when you are very angry with someone and know that you will get very adverse reactions if you tell him/her this, instead of expressing your feelings, you can stop yourself from expressing them by contracting your throat and holding your breath, or you can retroflect and hold your feelings in by clenching your teeth or fists and crossing your arms; in the same way, even though you want to hit the person, you can dig your nails into your palms, bite your lips or nails, hit yourself or even tear your hair out. In the beginning, these acts are done consciously in response to a particular situation or person. However, if these acts become a habit, if they become chronic and occur unconsciously, then a conflict emerges between the muscles that allow these actions and those that work in just the opposite direction, and the energy is blocked. In time, the person not only forgets the reasons for such reactions such as why he/she has clenched fists, but he/she might even be unaware of the fact that his/her fists are clenched. However, whether he/she is doing it consciously or not, he/she will keep on doing this.

People who frequently use the retroflection style of contact suffer in particular from muscular-skeletal problems (Zinker 1977, 103). Tension in the neck, shoulders, and arms and chest pains are typical for them.

This conflict emerging in the muscles due to the polarities such as do/ don't, stop/act, yes/no eventually affects the body posture (Perls et al. 1951/1996, 162–164). For example, when the pelvic region is tensed, flexible movement of the upper body, arms, and the head is prevented. Kepner (1987, 151) has indicated that chronic retroflection could affect (a) muscle development, (b) posture, by causing certain parts of the body to lean forward, backward, right, or left, and (c) distribution of body fat. He has claimed that, just like the excess accumulation of sediments where a river flows slowly, chronic deficiency of blood circulation and energy flow at muscle joints will lead to accumulation of fat in those regions.

According to the Gestalt approach, body, feelings, and mind work as a whole. Hence, emotional and intellectual characteristics play a role in the emergence of physical disturbances. Starting from this viewpoint, Sills et al. (1998, 66) have noted that retroflected sadness can manifest itself as a cold (because of streaming eyes and nose), retroflected anger as ulceration (because of the stomach acids), and retroflected fear as high fever. Chronic retroflection can also cause psychogenic headaches (Perls et al. 1951/1996, 166). For example, when somebody hurts your feelings or makes you angry, you might want to cry. However, if you believe that others should not see you crying because this is a sign of weakness, you might try to stop yourself from crying by tensing and squeezing your head muscles. In this case, even though what you really want is to squeeze the head of the person who put you in this situation, you retroflect your hurt or anger by tensing your head and giving yourself a headache. Hence, in retroflection, the person who is aching and the one causing the ache is actually one and the same. Another way of preventing crying is tensing the diaphragm muscles. In this case, you will be retroflecting your hurt or anger onto your stomach.

One of the most important retroflection-related physical symptoms is holding the breath (Perls et al. 1951/1996, 168). Holding the breath not only prevents the experiencing of feelings and senses but also prevents converting them into sounds and words since while you are holding your breath, it is impossible to make any sound. When breath holding becomes a chronic habit, it is impossible to be aware of your feelings, your rib cage becomes narrowed, your back arches, and your shoulders close up in a forward position. Consequently, now you have retroflected all your feelings and hold them within yourself.

How to Work with Retroflection in Therapy

The purpose of working with retroflection during therapy is to change the direction of retroflected behavior and to direct it toward the right target. During this work, in the beginning, by giving attention to what and how the client is retroflecting, the client's contact with him/herself is established and then the efforts toward directing the retroflection to the environment are supported (Polster and Polster 1974, 87). In this way, the obstructed need is revealed, expressed, and met, and thus satisfaction is achieved.

There are certain points that should be taken into consideration during work on directing retroflection at the environment. First of all, the person has to become aware of and accept feelings such as anger, sexuality, sadness, and even love and excitement that he or she has so far not been able to express in his/her environment, and this is no easy task because the person has not been in contact with his or her feelings for a very long time. To be aware of such feelings and to accept them can lead to the emergence of feelings such as anxiety, fear, shame, or guilt, which are hard to deal with and hence can cause resistance. Therefore, before starting the work on directing the retroflection at the environment, the therapist should support the client sufficiently to enable him or her to deal with these feelings such as anxiety, fear, shame, or guilt and to overcome his or her resistance.

Some people are extremely disturbed and even feel horrified about being aware of their anger (Perls et al. 1951/1996, 166). For such people, it is not possible to accept that they are angry with their parents, authority, faith, or God. Consequently, rather than show their anger to others, they prefer to live by retroflecting it, as in this way, they receive some satisfaction, albeit partial. When a person is angry with him/herself instead of others, he/she can at least experience his/her anger in a primitive, undistinguished, and rough way. Otherwise, he/she would have no way at all to experience this anger. Those who retroflect their anger think, "I had better get angry with myself rather than others, this at least will not harm anybody." Obviously harming the self causes less guilt than harming others. However, even though the anger has been retroflected, since the person is actually angry with someone else, this reflects on his/her relations with the other person and prevents contact.

On the other hand, when seen from a clinical perspective, anger is highly beneficial and even necessary for the emergence of happiness and creativity (Perls et al. 1951/1996, 176–179). Furthermore, reversing the retroflection of anger does not mean creating an anger that did not previously exist. The person is already angry. If the person is able to accept his/her anger and the need to express this, then he/she can direct it at the environment in a healthier and mature way. The next step in therapy is for the person to be aware of those needs that cause anger and to determine constructive ways of meeting them. Otherwise, whether the anger is retroflected or directed at the environment, the person will not be able to establish healthy contact with his/her environment and will be unhappy.

While working on what and how the person is retroflecting, one of the methods that can be used is investigating his or her attitudes toward him/herself (Perls et al. 1951/1996, 154–158). To facilitate this, the therapist can make use of various questions, the client's narratives, and his or her bodily and non-verbal reactions during the therapy. Therapist can seek answers to the following questions in order to be able to define what and how the client was retroflecting:

How is the client punishing him/herself?

Whom does the client actually want to punish?

Does he/she exhibit self-harming behavior?

Whom does the client actually want to harm?

How does the client want to inflict this harm?

Is the client self-pitying?

From whom does he/she want to receive pity?

In what areas does the client expect to be perfect?

In what areas does the client want others to be perfect?

In what areas does the client not trust him/herself?

Whom and in what areas does the client want to trust?

Whom does he/she want to trust him/her?

To whom can the client not say "no"?

Whom does the client not want to say "no" to him/her?

Maybe you would like to answer these questions and become aware of what you are retroflecting. So, take a paper and pen and try it.

Another method that can be followed in defining retroflection is to increase bodily awareness. For example, if the client wraps his/her arms around him/herself while talking about something during therapy, the therapist could first help him/her to understand what he/she is doing, then explore what this means and then could ask, "Who do you actually want to hug?" or "Whose hugs do you need?" Or, when a client talks with clenched fists, the question of whom he/she wants to hit could be raised. In particular, when the therapist notices the client is holding his or her breath, the focus could then fall on this, and an investigation could be made into what the client may be holding in: tears, shouts, the desire to run away, violence, love, laughter, and compassion, whatever it may be. Moreover, when the client mentions physical symptoms such as pain, a burning sensation, tension, or pressure, work could be carried out on what they mean for the person. While working with these types of physical symptoms, the best way to follow is to focus on the symptoms and, by asking the person to exaggerate them, to help the client to be aware of the affected muscle groups related with his/her physical symptoms. The ways and means of working with the bodily and nonverbal reactions of the client during therapy are given in detail in the section on body language.

Once the person becomes aware of what and how he/she is retroflecting physically, then comes the stage of directing the retroflection at the environment, that is, toward actual people or situations. For example, a client may feel a pain in the throat and numbness in the hands while talking about a friend. While working on these physical symptoms, it might become clear that the pain in the throat is preventing the patient from shouting and the numbness in the hands prevents their movement, or in other words, the pain in the throat is the retroflection of a desire to shout and the numbness is the retroflection of a desire to hit out. Obviously, in such a case, the client cannot be asked to find the friend and start punching him/her while shouting just for the sake of directing his/her retroflection at the environment, but he/she can be asked to orient his/her anger toward a pillow. In the Gestalt approach, pillows are very often used while working on retroflection. Hence, each Gestalt therapist has to have a number of pillows of different sizes in his/her office. What is important during this practice is to have the person be able to express his/her feelings with sounds and words while trying to punch the pillow at the same time, i.e., to manage both simultaneously.

Another point that is important in terms of the reversal of retroflection is for the person to be aware of whose substitute the pillow is while expressing his/her feelings verbally and bodily. In other words, the client should know with whom he/she is angry with and at whom he/she is shouting and expressing violence. Otherwise merely being angry, shouting, hitting out, or similar manifestations of feelings will not be very helpful in reversing the retroflection.

In conclusion, the first step in work related to the retroflection style of contact during therapy is defining what is retroflected and how. Later, for the reversal of the retroflection, the work will be carried on directing and expressing the feelings of the person and the needs underlying them to the environment and the correct targets. Through such work, it becomes possible for the blocked energy of the person to be usable again and hence to have the person mobilized toward his/her desires and needs.

13

EGOTISM

What Is Egotism?

The first person to mention egotism as a style of contact was Goodman (referred to in Wheeler 1998, 82). According to Goodman, egotism occurs when a person, instead of experiencing a situation, watches the experiencing self and the environmental factors from a distance. In other words, egotism is the process of self-monitoring or "spectatoring" (Sills et al. 1998, 67).

A person who uses egotism as a style of contact, instead of establishing contact with other people or the environment, watches the contacting self. For example, while walking on the street, if instead of paying attention to the street on which you are walking—to the traffic lights, shop windows, and so on—you are focusing on how you are walking, how you look, who is looking at you, and whether or not your clothes suit you, then you are watching yourself. When you are dining out with your boy-/girlfriend, instead of being aware of the physical environment you are in, enjoying the meal, listening to the music, and having a naturally flowing conversation with your partner, if you are focusing on how you look, how you are positioning your hands and arms, and what you should be saying, again you are watching yourself.

In a similar way, during lovemaking, to engage in thoughts such as, "Do I look beautiful or handsome?" "What should I do now?" "Does he find me too passive?" is another example of egotism.

According to the Gestalt approach, the contact boundary is the point where the self and others meet. However, in egotism, there are not two people meeting at the contact boundary but just one person actually meeting him/herself. Hence, as there is no mutual relationship, the person is relating only to the self. The self-observing person is so busy with his/her thoughts, behaviors, and feelings that he/she is not even aware of whom or what he/she is encountering (Latner 1992, 40). Since the person is unaware of what is going on in the environment, he/she is only involved with him/herself and the impression he/she makes on others. This involvement can be positive, as with self-admiration, self-congratulation, or self-appreciation, as well as negative in cases of self-criticism or self-humiliation (Joyce and Sills 2003, 123). Whether positive or negative, the person comments on or judges everything he/she does or does not do or say. For example, Richard, when having tea with his colleagues at work, instead of enjoying the tea he was drinking, was observing and judging himself drinking tea with thoughts such as "I feel so tense, I am sure everybody can see this, God knows what they think about me," or "I am done if they see my hands shaking, everybody will think what a stupid person I am." As can be seen here, we have fantasies and thoughts based on egotism (Philippson 2001, 96). Obviously all of us have met people who are very quiet, who cannot find anything to say and thus give an impression of being cold, or we have been together with people who love talking about themselves, who try to prove to others how smart, successful, or good they are. All these behaviors are products of egotism.

One of the conditions for contact is to let oneself go. To achieve this, a person should be able to take risks and be ready for new situations and relationships. According to Laura Perls (1992), only if we can let ourselves go can we enjoy something we have experienced and have the chance of learning something from it (referred to in Sills et. al. 1998, 68). However, egotism hinders letting go as the person is continuously preoccupied with how he/she looks from outside and what people are thinking about him/her. This prevents the person from being spontaneous and causes him/her to be cautious and well- advised all the time (Wheeler 1998, 82). The person who is engaged in self-observation, or egotism, needs to control him/herself all the time. For the sake of not making a mistake, not looking like a fool, or not to be ridiculous, the person freezes and cannot mobilize. In egotism, the person needs to control not only him/herself but other people and the environmental conditions as well (Crocker 1999, 94). Such a person never wants to be faced with surprises and situations calling for risk taking. The opposite of egotism is impulsivity.

The Advantages and Disadvantages of Egotism

In some instances, egotism is beneficial and even necessary. For example, for a person who has just started to drive, for a therapist who wants to develop his/her skills by listening to a taped interview, or for an actor who is rehearsing a role in front of a mirror, using egotism as a way of contact is highly advantageous. Egotism is also useful in terms of the awareness work often used in the Gestalt approach. During this work, to have the client observe him/herself can help the person to become aware of what and how he/she is doing and what and how he/she should change.

According to Goodman, egotism is a process required in order to overcome hardships and achieve maturity (referred to in Crocker 1999, 95). Egotism enables a person to confront the difficulties he/she faces and ensures perseverance. In other words, egotism enables the person to be prepared for the situations to be encountered and to reach goals whose achievement requires considerable time. Perls et al. (1951/1969, 456) have also stated that egotism is a necessary step in preventing hasty decision making and the pattern of "do-undo." One of the most characteristic features of egotism is that it slows down the person, and this prevents him/her from committing to act in a rush that will be regretted later (Clarkson and Mackewn 1993, 77). In certain other situations, by preventing impulsive reacting, it allows the person to make contact in a more healthy way (Philippson 2001, 96). Egotism, at the same time, makes the person more attentive to his/her self-care and more respectful toward the rights and ideas of others. Those who are always starting fights and who mistreat others are people who never use egotism as a style of contact.

Through egotism, the person tries to save him/herself from getting hurt, wounded, or upset, but frequently using this style of contact also prevents spontaneity and causes the person to be alienated from him/herself and the environment (Clarkson 1991, 51). Self-observing during contact prevents him/her giving something to or receiving something from the other person. If the person is trying to control the surprises or those things that cannot be controlled in life—that is, if he/she cannot let go through being self-aware and vigilant all the time, then he/she cannot forge healthy contact, and the harmony between the self and the environment is disrupted. For example, egotism lies at the root of many sexual dysfunctions. People who suffer from sexual dysfunctions, instead of enjoying their sexuality, are as if watching themselves during lovemaking. This, however, prevents both the brain from making the necessary preparations for sex and the body from giving appropriate responses, and this makes it impossible for the person to reach sexual satisfaction.

Continuous self-control and failure to let oneself go prevents the person from feeling complete or fully satisfied in many areas (Perls et al. 1951/1969, 456). For example, a person who tries to be aware of everything he/she is doing, that is, self-observing, might be thinking in conversation with a friend, "Right now I am looking at her and smiling. Now I raised my eyebrows. My friend must be wondering why I did it. Now I asked her what happened next, and I was a little loud." In a conversation carried out in this vein, the person finds it very difficult to give the appropriate reactions to the other and may not even remember what the other person has said. Consequently, nothing comes out of such a conversation. The extreme self-awareness of the person, the constant preoccupation of the brain with the inner voice, thoughts, plans, and fantasies can even lead to a schizoid withdrawal (Philippson 2001, 96). Egotism also plays an important role in anxiety disorders, phobias, and obsessive-compulsive disorders. Chronic use of egotism is also a significant characteristic of narcissist personality disorder (Yontef 1993, 428).

The Basis of Egotism

The most distinctive characteristic of the development of egotism as a style of contact is the overcritical approach of parents to children. In some families, the child is constantly watched, followed, and checked. Everything the child does or says is evaluated and remarked upon. In some families, there is no constant monitoring and control, but even the slightest negative behavior or "failure" of the child is never missed. It is talked about immediately and even exaggerated. In such families, parents show reactions such as "What a dirty child you are, nobody plays with dirty children," when the child dirties his/her clothes while playing in the garden, "How stupid you are, nobody is going to like you," when an exam is failed, or "You are scruffy and inconsiderate, you are giving me a bad time," when the child spreads out his/her toys while playing. Reactions of this type cause the child to introject messages such as "I will not be accepted as I am" and "In order to be liked and appreciated and to get attention, I have to be perfect all the time, everywhere, and in everything." Not only the frequent and negative criticisms but also exaggerated positive messages play a role in the development of egotism. For example, remarks such as "You are so pretty, there is no one prettier than you," "You are so smart, you can do anything," or "You are such a good child that you always consider and never irritate me," just like the adverse remarks, give the child a message to be perfect all the time, everywhere, and in everything. Furthermore such exaggerated praise causes the child to see him/herself as superior to others and so to judge his/her friends. Another attitude that causes egotism is to constantly compare the child with his/her siblings, the children of neighbors, relatives, or friends. Open statements such as "Look how smart your brother is, he is always getting high grades," "How great other people's children are and just look at yourself," or insinuations such as "She is such a well-behaved child, I love her very much," "He is such a successful child, his family must be proud of him" also make the child feel inadequate. In the end, a child who is brought up in this atmosphere becomes an adult who constantly compares him/herself with others, who always believes that others are better, and who fears that, because of any small mistake, he/she will not be liked or appreciated. All this, while creating a need to constantly control the self and the environment at the same time, leads to a tendency constantly to judge the self and others. At the bottom of this is the fact that the person sees him/herself either lower or higher than the others but in either case not feeling secure.

Personality Characteristics of People Who Use Egotism as a Contact Style Frequently

The people who frequently use egotism are tense, anxious, controlled, introvert, shy, skeptical, and slow individuals. Their self-confidence is low, and they are not able to empathize. Such people give too much importance to their environment. They cannot tolerate even the possibility of being criticized by the people they do not know. As they are always preoccupied with others' opinions of themselves, they cannot establish warm or sincere relationships. Even if they seem warm and friendly, because they believe this is how they should be, they actually do not feel this way. They are not alive, active, and joyous. Since they are always vigilant and careful, they cannot give spontaneous reactions. They try to be excellent in almost everything, and because of this, they cannot achieve satisfaction from what they do. As they cannot accept themselves as they are and as they believe that they always have to be the best, prettiest, or most successful, they cannot integrate and assimilate the characteristics they have, and these sit upon them like a new suit of unfamiliar shape and proportions (Clarkson 1991, 55). Some people who frequently use egotism are very pleased with themselves and indulge in self-admiration in a narcissistic way. These people, due to their lack of empathy and grandiose feelings, look down on others and are oversensitive to criticism (Yontef 1988).

In families where egotism is frequently used, rules are very important. Family members, rather than doing what they want, do what is regarded as right and reasonable. In such families, the concepts of shame and sin are significant. As they are highly judgmental and intolerant, the family members display a hostile and aggressive attitude toward each other. They are not very talkative, and hence, they cannot solve problems as there is little or no contact with each other. They give much attention to making plans and programs and hence they dislike sudden occurrences or surprises. Their decision making takes a very long time, and even then, they are still not sure about their decisions. The family members are very limited, rigid, and superficial, not only among themselves, but also in their contacts with their environment.

How to Work with Egotism in Therapy

The purpose of work carried out on egotism during therapy is to help the person establish satisfactory contact with others and the environment by moderating his/her egotism. To this end, the initial work is designed to draw attention to the moments that the client stops the I-Thou dialogue and turns inward and, by sharing this observation with the client, to bring him/her back to the here and now (Joyce and Sills 2003, 123). For example, if during therapy the client suddenly stops when talking on a subject and says, "My heart has started pounding, do you hear it?" and keeps repeating the same thing without paying any attention to what the therapist is saying, then keeps silent for a long time, or skips the details of the subject under discussion, then whether egotism is involved should be explored. The therapist should also question the relations of the client with his/her family, friends, and people in the environment to investigate whether or not egotism is being used as a style of contact in his/her everyday life.

Once the client becomes aware of the fact that he/she is self-observing instead of establishing contact, then work can start on what he/she is feeling at that moment and what his/her thoughts are. For example, during a session, Sue explained how, attending a meeting of her relatives, tense and anxious she felt even though she knew many people there, how she sat by herself in a distant corner of the room almost without talking with anybody, and left early. While the causes of her tension and anxiety were being explored, it became evident that during the meeting, she kept thinking, "I wonder if my outfit is appropriate?" "Did I put too much food on my plate?" "I am sure everybody is aware of how tense I am and has figured out that I am troubled." Todd talked about not going out to lunch with his colleagues because of thoughts such as "Will I blush if I talk?" "Will my voice falter?" and "Can I find something interesting to talk about?" and how this made him feel bad. Once the underlying feelings and thoughts of egotism as a style of contact are defined, the two-chair technique can be used to have the client recount his/her feelings, thoughts, and wishes to one of the people who were there. During such an experiment, Todd chose to express his feelings and thoughts to Mike, to whom he felt closer than the others. Sue decided to share her feelings, thoughts, and wishes with her aunt by marriage with whom she felt more comfortable. During the exercise, Sue told her aunt how alone and tense she felt there, and then asked her aunt to talk and pay attention to her. Then, taking the aunt's place she talked to herself.

During this dialogue, while Sue was sharing her feelings and thoughts with her aunt, she realized that it was easier for her than she had expected, that she felt better after expressing herself, and that as her aunt, she felt closer to Sue after hearing about Sue's sharing herself. During the next stage of therapy, the client was helped to develop alternative ways to achieve her wishes. For example, during the exercise, Sue defined three alternatives in order to actualize her wish about having her aunt talk with her and pay her attention: (a) to go to her aunt without waiting for her to come, (b) to initiate the conversation by asking how she is and how her children are, (c) to discuss what she has been doing recently and particularly to talk about the places she went on holiday. Following the determination of alternatives, the client could be asked to imagine those alternative ways as if he/she were doing them in the here and now and to explain what is happening and how he/she is feeling in the imagination in the present tense or to act them out in the session.

Another point that should be taken into consideration during therapy is to help the client in focusing his/her attention away from him/herself and onto other persons and the environment. For this purpose, imagination and awareness exercises can be utilized. For example, it might be suggested to the client to once again remember that particular meeting and visualize the place it was held, what the other people were wearing, doing, eating, talking about, and what they might have been feeling. As people who use egotism as a style of contact are frequently, if not constantly, preoccupied with themselves, they might find it very difficult to remember the characteristics of others. In such cases, they can be asked to make observations in their daily lives about others and to talk about those observations in the following sessions.

In some cases the purpose could be not the prevention of the self-observation of the clients but to make them learn how to do it. For example, in one session, Patricia talked about her son's excess weight, how angry this made her, and how it was ruining his health as well as his appearance. She added that she felt justified in being angry with him, sometimes she couldn't stop herself and even hit him, but everything she did was for his own good. Patricia was so involved with her own feelings and thoughts that she was not paying any attention to what her son was thinking, feeling, or what he wanted. Then Patricia was asked to enter a dialogue with her son through a two-chair experiment on his eating problems. The dialogue developed like this:

Patricia (as herself):	*Look, my love, don't eat so much. It is so bad for your health. Furthermore they will laugh at you because of it. Why should you eat so much? I love you very much, and I don't want you to be hurt. The other day they were shouting "Fatso" after you.*
Therapist:	*Now take your son's place, and as your son, tell your mother what you feel when she talks like this.*
Patricia (as her son):	*All right, Mother, I won't eat too much again. I will not eat ice cream and chocolates.*
Therapist:	*Tell your mother what you are feeling.*
Patricia (as her son):	*OK, Mother, I will be more careful.*
Therapist:	*Don't tell your mother what you are going to do. Tell her about your feelings. Are you sorry? Are you angry? Are you happy with what you just heard?*
Patricia (as her son):	*I regret all I have done. I am sorry.*

(At this stage, Patricia was still not aware of what her son's feelings were. When she took her son's place, she said those things that she wanted to hear from him and what she wanted him to feel.)

Therapist:	*You are feeling sorry and regretful for the things that you have done. But tell your mother what her words, her expressions make you feel.*
Patricia (as her son):	*You want what is best for me and I am making you angry. I am angry with myself. I don't like myself. You don't love me either, you dislike me. I annoy you. I am so ugly.*

At this point, Patricia started to sob. Later she realized that as a child she was also rather overweight, and now she was getting angry with her son just as her mother had been with her. She remembered how her mother's negative remarks about her weight used to make her very sad and angry and how these feelings made her want to eat even more. Remembering this helped her to realize what her son could be feeling because of her comments and actions and how she was actually teaching him egotism. Later on in the dialogue, she apologized for the things she had said and done to him and eventually started to be much more sensitive toward his feelings and needs. Another important aspect that became apparent during this dialogue was Patricia's realization of the unfinished business she had with her mother. While working with egotism, unfinished business comes up quite often. Hence, work should be carried out during therapy on the completion of unfinished business and changing the introjections that lie at the base of egotism.

At the end of work carried out on egotism, it will be possible for the person to establish contact with others (a) without feeling anxious and fearful and in a spontaneous and sincere way, (b) to care for others as much as him/herself during contact, (c) to feel neither superior nor inferior to them, and (d) to accept him/herself and the others as they are.

14

CONFLUENCE

What Is Confluence?

Confluence is a state where the person and the environment cannot be distinguished from each other (Clarkson 1991, 55). Contact is necessary for growth and development (Korb et al. 1989, 39). Just as plants need contact with earth, water, and air in order to grow and develop, similarly humans need contact with each other and their environment. Contact, indeed, occurs at the boundary between the person and the environment. Perls (1973, 38) explained this through the following example: We are composed of millions of cells. If these cells were in confluence with each other, then we could not function as a whole organism. All cells are separated from one other by porous membranes, which are the places where what is to be accepted within the membrane and what is to be rejected are determined, that is to say, where contact or differentiation occurs. If the different parts of our bodies were not functioning both as part of a whole and as unique to themselves, that is, if they were in confluence, then none could fulfill its own function. Similarly, there needs to be a differentiation, a boundary between people and their environment, so that they can both realize their own functions and can grow and develop by contacting each other. According to the Gestalt approach, having no boundary between the person and others is called confluence.

Confluence can be experienced in many different ways. For example, when we have eaten something, then we cannot differentiate between ourselves and that food: it has become part of us, and we are in confluence with it. Similarly, gaining new information on a subject could also be seen as an example of confluence. When you read something new and when you decide to keep this information in your mind and learn it, it becomes knowledge that belongs to you, and it merges with what you already know (Perls et al. 1951/1996, 119). Newborn babies live in confluence with their mothers; they are not aware of the differences between their inner or environmental stimuli or between themselves and the others. Confluence can be seen in situations where a person is either overly cautious or drunk with joy. Clarkson (1991, 55) drew attention to how a feeling of disappearance of boundaries is experienced during creative activities or meditation. People could also be in confluence with religious institutions, clubs, or professional associations. For example, fanatical fans of a football team, as they are in confluence with the team they are supporting, react to the actions of the players of the opposing team or the referee as if they were directed at them in person. Some people are in confluence with their job. They work very long hours, and even when they are not working, they think about it. They evaluate themselves in terms of their work and feel good only when the work is going well. Others are in confluence with their homes. Such people are very uneasy if their homes are a little untidy or dirty and even feel as if they are also lacking in tidiness and cleanliness.

Some other people are in confluence with society. They cannot see themselves as separate individuals and seem as if they have melted and disappeared within social beliefs, attitudes, value judgments, and rules. Still others are merged with another person. People who are in confluence with society or a person are so merged with them that they are not aware of their own thoughts, feelings, desires, or even their bodies. Those who say, "I give great value to what others are saying" or "We never go anywhere without each other, we do everything together," those who think others will make better decisions on their behalf, those who claim to be very devoted to their child, mother, boyfriend or friend, are in a state of confluence. At the base of the need for confluence is the fear of not being loved or appreciated or of being abandoned (Clarkson 1991, 78). Because of these fears, the person is as if stuck to another person or group. The other extreme of confluence is isolation (Yontef 1993, 142), where the boundary between the individual and the others is so thick and rigid that contact is impossible. The fear of "being swallowed up" or "hemmed in" by others lies at the root of isolation.

The Advantages and Disadvantages of Confluence

Confluence is a style of contact we experience especially with our loved ones. For example, falling in love is a type of experience totally based on confluence. Just as we were dependent on our mothers for survival during our confluence stage with her, when we are in love, we think that we cannot live without our lover. Just as we were unhappy as a baby when we could not see our mother or hear her voice, we are also unhappy when we do not see our lover and reach for the phone to at least hear his/her voice. If this is not convenient, we send a message to be sure of his/her existence. Confluence can emerge not only in this romantic love but in all types of relationships that involve loving. Confluence gives the person a sense of belonging and being safe (Polster and Polster 1974, 75). It is also useful in enabling people to approach each other with empathy and to understand the feelings of others. Furthermore, such experiences make us feel loved, appreciated, and valued. A person who is confluent with society feels successful and good when he/she observes the rules of society and is happy. Confluence can also be considered as a style of contact that protects us from facing feelings such as loneliness or emptiness that create existential anxieties (Clarkson 1991, 56–57).

Healthy relations have a rhythm. People approach each other spontaneously as the situation demands, move away, and then again approach and move away. Once real contact is established, the experienced confluence is very healthy and satisfying and is followed by wandering away. For example, a baby is in confluence with his/her mother during breast-feeding. When the baby is full, he/she lets go of the mother's breast happily and moves away from the mother. After a while, when he/she is hungry again or needs to feel the warmth of the mother, the baby once again wants to be in confluence with the mother. Confluence can be an essential part of what Maslow (1962) calls the "peak experience," a moment of "highest happiness and satisfaction" (referred to in Korb et al. 1989, 60). In such a situation, the person is only interested in what has led to this peak experience, has integrated with it, and there is nothing to fear or react against. One of the best examples of such a moment of integration is sexual intercourse. Confluence is a very rich experience. I-Thou relationship experienced during therapy can sometimes have such a characteristic. This kind of peak experience cannot be preplanned or deliberately arranged and does not last long. After a while, the peak experience is completed, and in order to experience confluence again, people have to move away and separate from each other for some time. In this way, it is possible to enjoy a healthy life in a balance, where our common needs are met through confluence and our personal needs by differentiation and moving away.

If confluence becomes permanent, then it becomes harmful. This means that, since the person cannot move away from whom or what he/she has merged with, then there will be no opportunity to come together once more and to establish contact. Just as we cannot feel our hand after holding hands for a long time, when we stay in a state of confluence for an extended period of time, we can no longer feel each other and hence become unable to establish contact. As contact is not possible in the state of confluence, no new figure can be formed, and consequently, there is no excitement (Perls et al. 1951/1996, 118). Such a relationship continues in a monotonous, boring, static, and insensitive way until the person who wants to get away from the state of confluence puts an end to it. In general, these ending are very sudden and traumatic. For example, statements such as "We never argued, I can't understand why he left me," "We were fine one day, and the next day, she called and broke it off," or "He was a very respectful and quiet child, never talked back to me; why did he try to commit suicide?" are indicators of confluence.

People who have merged with society, on the other hand, cannot fulfill their own desires, feelings, and needs as they are constantly striving to keep the rules, to be liked by everybody, and to try to do good deeds for all. Instead of shaping the situation according to themselves, they shape themselves according to the situation. They have a constant need for people who will end their worries and who will openly approve of them. Confluence can cause a person to be stuck with a certain thought, situation or feeling. Such people, instead of developing new modes of behavior, thoughts, habits, and solutions, take no risks at all and hold on to old familiar rules, people, and situations (Perls et al. 1951/1996, 145). Consequently they feel chronically frustrated or become depressed.

Chronic confluence puts a person into a state where he/she does not know what he/she wants to do and what prevents him/her from doing it. For example, let us assume that in various instances you wanted to cry, but believing that it is a sign of weakness prevented yourself from crying by contracting the muscles of your diaphragm. This contraction, which you at first did deliberately, may in time become a habit, and you start to contract those muscles unconsciously whenever you feel like crying. Consequently, the need to breathe and to cry is in confluence. Contracting the diaphragm muscles makes you hold your breath. Eventually you become a person who can neither breathe easily and regularly nor cry. As you cannot cry, you cannot show your unhappiness and, after a while, cannot even remember what made you unhappy. Perls (1973, 40) has stated that the habit of preventing crying by holding the breath in particular, if employed for a long time, may lead to asthma, and this type of confluence could be playing a role in various psychosomatic illnesses.

One of the harmful cases of confluence is the mother's inability to come out of merging with her child for an extended time, thus failing to meet her own needs as she tries to meet those of the child and eventually becoming depressed or starting to have serious problems with her spouse. Confluence is a very frequently used style of contact particularly in borderline personality disorders. Those with such disorders can merge with a person whom they have overidealized, or they can be in confluence with someone they devaluate (Clarkson 1991, 57).

The items related with confluence on the Revised Gestalt Contact Styles Questionnaire, which was confirmed as reliable and valid by Aktaş and Daş (2002), are given below. Would you like to mark the items and find out how often you use confluence as a style of contact?

After reading each point, circle the letter that best reflects your status. The meaning of each letter is as follows:

A: Quite appropriate for me

B: Appropriate for me

C: I am undecided

D: Not generally appropriate for me

E: Not appropriate for me at all

1.	I get along well with almost everybody.	A B C D E
2.	I live according to the expectations of my family.	A B C D E
3.	When people get serious, I try to lighten the atmosphere.	A B C D E
4.	My behavior is polite and refined.	A B C D E
5.	Self-control is important for me.	A B C D E
6.	I talk as if I am apologizing.	A B C D E
7.	I don't easily become angry.	A B C D E
8.	I expect people to be tolerant of each other's differences.	A B C D E
9.	I am not easily convinced.	A B C D E
10.	I find it difficult to say no to those who are close to me.	A B C D E
11.	I like to get away from obstinate people I am with.	A B C D E
12.	I prefer roundabout ways rather than reacting directly.	A B C D E
13.	I obey the wishes of others.	A B C D E

The scores of the items are A=5, B=4, C=3, D=2, E=1. Only in items 9 and 11 is a reverse scoring used. That is, for those items the scoring is thus A=1, B=2, C=3, D=4, E=5. Thus, the maximum score you can get is 65. The higher your score is, the more you use confluence as a style of contact.

The Basis of Confluence

At the root of confluence lies the fact that parents regard their children not as different individuals but as extensions or even as copies of themselves. According to these parents, the child "belongs" to them, and consequently, it is obvious that it is the parents, not the child, who will decide what and how he/she is going to do, think and feel, as well as what his/her needs are. Parents who contact their children through confluence can never tolerate the individualization and differentiation of their children (Perls 1973, 40). In such families, the children are expected to meet all demands of the parents in the exact way and time they want. These parents want their children to completely merge with them; they do whatever they can to accomplish this. If the child is in confluence with them, then he/she is approved, supported, and protected. If the child is insistent about those demands, behaviors and feelings that the parents do not approve; that is, if the child refuses to be confluent with them, then he/she is immediately punished with insults, being sent away, and even violence. "I don't like naughty children," "If you behave like that, then you are not my son," and "If you loved me, you would fulfill my every demand" are frequently used statements in such homes. It is obvious that, hearing these things, the children, who need the love and attention of their parents, have no other choice but to enter confluence with them. Eventually such children learn to completely give up their own desires and needs and cannot even imagine that they could have desires and needs of their own. These parents cannot tolerate those traits, actions, and needs of their children that are different from theirs. Particularly in some cultures where "no matter how old you are, you are still our child" is the prevalent mentality, the parents try to control the life of their children even if they are holding down jobs, are married, or they themselves become parents. They cannot accept the fact that their children are adults and cannot give up being confluent with them. One day, a father telephoned me and said, "I want to bring my kid to you, he just does not behave as I wish him to behave. I will disown him, but maybe you can put some sense in him and make him behave as I want." The "kid" mentioned on the phone was a thirty-four-year-old married engineer.

In the learning of confluence as a style of contact, not only the family, but also the value judgments of society play a part. Societies that are more conservative, bound with rules, strictly devoted to traditions, and do not place importance on individuality raise people who are not aware of their desires, thoughts, and needs, who do not take responsibility for them, and who expect solutions to come from others. What is important for such people is whether or not the others approve of what they are doing. They do everything that they assume that society expects from them and believe that consequently they will be successful, well-esteemed, famous, free from disease, and untroubled by personal difficulties (Polster and Polster 1974, 95). As they are not even aware of whether or not they really want to do what they are doing, they do not enjoy it. They focus on the result rather than the process. They try to abide by rules set by someone unknown and to make efforts without knowing who they will be pleasing. Hence, when these efforts do not bring the expected results, they do not know with whom to be angry either. These people, who are accused by others of not showing enough effort, not working hard enough, or not behaving in such and such a manner, continue to try to do the best they can. Unfortunately, by the time they understand that no matter what they do, they cannot please everybody, they have reached the end of their lives.

Personality Characteristics of People Who Use Confluence as a Style of Contact Frequently

Those who use confluence as a style of contact are generally well-adjusted people with whom it is easy to establish contact (Kepner 1982). They have an extreme aversion to disagreement and conflict. When they do not agree with those around them, they assume that they will hurt them and worry intensely about this. For that reason, even when they are against the decision taken or what is to be done, they act as if they agree with the others. People who try to establish contact through confluence have great difficulty in saying "no" to others. Consequently, by choosing to say "yes" all the time, they try to cover up disagreements. They prefer to assume a humble attitude by not considering their own thoughts, feelings, and needs and thus perpetually play the role of victim. As they greatly fear conflict, their diplomatic skills are well developed. When the atmosphere of their surroundings becomes tense, they try to soften up the situation and look joyful. On the other hand, when their need for confluence is not met, they can try all possible ways to convince others, and if necessary, they do not hesitate to bribe or to bully (Perls et al. 1951/1996, 121).

People who need to be confluent lack self-confidence and cannot become individuals. Since they lack the power to support themselves in their relations, they fear rejection or abandonment (Zinker 1994, 125). Such people rather than indulging in a hard task such as searching for the meaning of their own desires, needs, and lives behave according to the demands of the people around them and allow others to determine the course of their lives (Polster and Polster 1974, 71). In a sense, they expect everything to fall into their laps with no effort on their part. They have no idea about when to terminate a situation or relationship and do not give up that person or situation even if they are unhappy or their expectations remain unfulfilled (Clarkson and Mackewn 1993, 75). New situations, new relations, new points of view are very scary for such people. Hence, they prefer to live without "rocking the boat" and, as far as possible, without changing anything.

In confluent families, all members are expected to agree on everything spontaneously and voluntarily (McConville 1995, 144). These families are proud of being in full agreement and enjoying the same things. They cannot tolerate differences in thoughts, feelings, and needs among the members. In such situations, they become very angry and do not feel safe. In these families where individual differences are not respected and where agreements cannot be reached because of individual differences, conflicts are frequent. They first try to convince each other, but when this is not possible, disagreements can turn into arguments, arguments into fights and fights into violence. Children, especially during adolescence, have great difficulties in this type of families.

Contact Patterns of People Who Frequently Use Confluence

Yontef (1993, 209) mentioned two types of contact patterns regarding confluence. In the first, both members of a couple are in confluence with each other, and as a couple, they separate themselves from their environment with a thick wall. It is as if they have abstracted themselves from society. In the second type, only one member of the couple has merged with the other by giving up his or her own desires, needs, and feelings.

In both contact patterns, there is a "three-legged race" arranged between two people who have decided to be always in agreement (Polster and Polster 1974, 93).

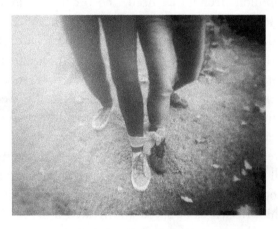

A three-legged race

This three-legged race emerges especially in love or husband-wife relations. One of the reasons for this is the individual's view regarding male-female relations. Some people, once they realize that they love each other and decide to be together, believe that from that moment on, they should do everything together and spend all their time in each other's company. They even think that their love for each other should take away their need for other people. Because of this, they distance themselves from their friends and hobbies and even neglect their schools or jobs. It is as if they have signed a pact always to be in agreement—to think, feel, and desire the same things. In the initial stages of the relationship, if it is not exaggerated, acting in accord with this approach may be fine. Just as the confluence in the mother-baby relationship is necessary and important for survival and growth of the baby, two lovers being confluent with each other can be beneficial—at least at the beginning—in ensuring the survival and growth of a fresh relationship. However, if this style of contact lasts for a long time, is exaggerated, and turns into a sticking together, then problems start to emerge. The approach-withdrawal rhythm that is essential for a good and healthy relationship becomes impaired. Such a relation can be an example of the above-mentioned first pattern type.

In the second pattern type, people behave not as two different individuals but as one. They use the pronoun "us" instead of "I" and are very happy with it. When one of the partners starts talking about a different opinion, feeling, or need, the other feels lonely and even abandoned (Joyce and Sills 2003, 121) The appearance of differences and boundaries is conceived as a threat to the relationship. In such cases, the basic feelings are anger and guilt (Polster and Polster 1974, 93). When one partner violates the confluence pact, that is, mentions a different desire or point of view, he/she feels guilty. Because of this feeling of guilt, the party apologizes for a demand that is not approved of by the other partner and gives up his/her wishes. Again, feeling guilty, he/she endures the rough behavior of the other and could even believe that it is well-deserved. The other person, when faced with a different demand or opinion from the partner, becomes very hurt and angry thinking of him/herself as betrayed and treated unfairly. While on one hand, he/she feels angry thinking how insensitive and indifferent the other person is; on the other hand, he/she starts feeling self-pity for being together with such a person. He or she progressively becomes more agitated and angry. In this type of relationship, even if the differences are initially ignored and not taken into consideration, eventually fights start. These fights are actually an indicator of the fact that they have started to contact, however, contact cannot be achieved because the powerful partner asserts his/her dominance, and the other one submits to this, and once again confluence is restored. In a relationship with a pattern of confluence, the powerful partner has a greater chance for self-expression and becoming an individual (Smith 1977, 224). The weaker partner, or the one who has a greater need for merging, while trying to avoid differences and misunderstandings, starts to feel hurt and angry and begins to be introversive. During disagreements, this partner either immediately accepts the opinions of the other without a full review of the situation and without expressing him/herself honestly or the same arguments go on and on with the problem left unsolved. In either case, contact totally disappears, and eventually, one partner, usually the more powerful, becomes fed up with the relationship.

Another case where this second pattern of confluence is often seen is in mother-child relations. Some mothers believe that they cannot be good mothers unless they sacrifice all and have decided to forget about their own needs, desires, and feelings and to think solely about their children. These mothers may be the ones who have first tried to merge with their husbands and, when that failed, turned to their children. Because of the nature of the relationship, as mothers are more powerful than their children, they expect them to obey their wishes in everything, and no matter how old they are, they want to control their lives. Within this pattern of confluence, while the children feel guilty for not fulfilling the wishes of their mother, they also feel angry for not getting what they want. In these relationships, mothers not only interfere with the daily relations of their children but also want to play an active role regarding their jobs and even in choosing their husbands or wives. This leads to even more serious problems with the male children and causes great conflicts in their marriages. The problems seen in marriages related with the wife and mother-in-law relations are caused by the competition between two women who want to be confluent with the same person. What is interesting is the fact that in such marriages both the wives and the mothers see the wish to be confluent with her husband/son as natural, but the conflict arises from different views about which of them has priority. Some families even do not even want their married children to be physically away and live in a far place or a different city.

How to Work with Confluence in Therapy

Those who use confluence frequently do not apply for therapy as long as they have a merged relationship. Their reason for coming to therapy is generally the significant problems they experience in their close relations. Applying for marriage therapy occurs only when one of the spouses decides to leave home or goes to court because the partner with a greater need for confluence does not believe that the relationship can end unless there is such a concrete reaction. When these couples come to therapy, they behave as if the partner who has given up on confluence is the guilty party.

The antidote to confluence is contact, differentiation, and the free expression of opinions (Polster and Polster 1974, 95). Hence, the purpose of therapy is to help the clients first to become aware of their own needs, feelings, and choices, then to make them realize that they can be loved, admired, and can survive despite their different sides from those around them and to gain the necessary power to support themselves. During therapy, whether or not a person has a tendency toward confluence can be detected from certain reactions. For example, if the client imitates how the therapist sits, tries to talk at the same speed as the therapist, and immediately agrees with what he/she says, then a tendency toward confluence should be investigated. Again, when a client talks only about positive, nice and good things or has difficulty in ending the session, this could be indicative of such a tendency. Similarly, a client's starting sentences with "us" or frequent use of expressions such as "everybody," "all the time," or "always" could also be indicators of confluence.

During therapy, in order to help the client become aware of his/her own wishes, needs, and feelings, the therapist frequently asks questions such as "What are you feeling just now?" "What do you want just now?" "What are you doing just now?" or "What do you need just now?" Care should be taken to ensure that the answers to these questions are specific and unique to the person. For example, it is important to convert answers such as "Everybody feels bad in such a situation" or "Everybody wants to be loved" into "I feel bad in such a situation" or "I want to be loved." To have the client express his/her personal feelings first to the therapist and then to the people he/she has difficulty in communicating with helps the client to get rid of confluent relations. Another point that should be taken into consideration during therapy is to emphasize the differences between the client and the person he/she is having difficulty in contacting, such as "I like to stay home and he likes to go out more," "In such cases while I feel lonely, he seems to be pleased with himself." The same type of work can also be carried out for similarities, such as "We both like to swim in the sea" or "We both love our mothers very much." The purpose of such practice is to help the client to see him/herself and the other person in their entirety, with all prevailing differences and similarities.

For a person who frequently uses confluence, giving it up and starting the process of individualization is rather hard and painful. As these people do not trust themselves and cannot take responsibility for living as an individual, they may initially try to merge with the therapist, and when this is not allowed, they may become angry. Therefore, in order to deal with confluence in therapy, it is necessary to establish a very strong trust relationship between the client and the therapist. Before starting to work on changing the confluence pattern, it is important for the person to fully realize the disadvantages of being confluent. Later, the client could be asked to talk about how he/she behaves in this confluent relation, and what he/she wants to achieve by behaving in this way. Then work is then carried out to make the client aware of whether or not he/she can achieve his/her goal in this way.

The feeling most often experienced by those who frequently use confluence is guilt—for feeling angry with people they love and for even thinking that they might feel anger. Actually, anger lies at the bottom of every feeling of guilt. The therapist should support the person so he/she can experience his/her anger without feeling guilty and later might invite the client to engage in pillow and empty-chair experiments in order to express his/her anger. However, the client should never be rushed, and such experiments should not be suggested before his/her self-support system is developed. Another practice that can be used during therapy is two-chair exercises where the person can have a dialogue with the person with whom he/she has merged. Such an exercise both helps the client to express him/herself to the other person better and also to see him/herself through the other person's eyes.

Below is a section from the dialogue Maggie had with her mother. Maggie is thirty-six years old, lives with her mother, and works in a public institution. She came to therapy with complaints of disinterest, lassitude, a frequent need to cry, oversleeping, and overeating. During the session, it was seen that Maggie was also experiencing serious relationship problems and was basically using confluence style of contact in her relations. Her mother was also an unhappy and lonely woman, and whenever Maggie wanted to do something by herself, to go out with her friends or to stay alone in her room, the mother confronted her with comments such as "My life is shortened because of you, why do you make me sad?" "You are leaving me alone, you will find me dead when you come home," or "Since you leave me alone, you don't love me, how ungrateful you are." Sometimes the mother would not talk to her for days.

Maggie (as her mother): *You are very ungrateful. I told you so many times about all the hardships I had while bringing you up. But you are selfish. All you care about is going out. Do you ever think about your mother?*

Maggie (as herself): *Mother, I only went to my friend's for some tea for two hours after work. What is wrong with this, for god's sake? You know that I work hard. Only yesterday I cleaned the whole house just because you wanted it. And also I took you to the movies the day before.*

Maggie (as her mother): *If I could, if I was able to do so, I would have cleaned the house. But I am sick, I can't lift a finger. I feel weak, I had so much hardship. I am not young like you.*

Maggie (as herself): *All right, Mother. I will not go out again. Are you satisfied now?*

Therapist: *Is this what you really want?*

Maggie (as herself): *No, but what can I do?*

Therapist: *Tell your feelings to your mother.*

Maggie (as herself): *Mother, I feel very bad when you are unhappy like this, but it is not possible for me to make you happy. No matter what I do, I can't satisfy you. I can't please you. Nothing is enough for you.*

Maggie (as her mother):	*I am aching all over, I am sick. I never had any good times to make me happy anyway. And what am I demanding from you? I want you to be with me after work. I am bored.*
Maggie (as herself):	*What else can you demand? I can't go anywhere. Even if I go, you keep calling me and ask, "When are you coming home?" Mother, I am thirty-six years old. When you were at my age, you were going out with my father and having a good time.*
Maggie (as her mother):	*Do you call it having a good time? I also had to take care of your sick aunt for years.*
Maggie (as herself):	(after a short silence, she started to cry) *I don't know what to say. It is no good.*
Therapist:	*Do you want to live her life? Those are her life conditions.*
Maggie (as herself):	*I just don't know* (started crying again), *but I don't want to make her sad.*
Therapist:	*All right, tell her this. Tell her, "Mother, in order not to make you sad, I will live your life. Since you took care of your husband's sister for years, now I will not go out either and will stay with you all the time!"*

When Maggie told this to her mother, she started laughing. The idea of not going out because her mother had taken care of her sister-in-law for years struck her as very funny. Later, she projected her anger against her mother toward the pillow and tried to develop different alternatives for their relationship.

Since the people who frequently use confluence generally find it difficult to say no, working on this might be worthwhile. Again using the two-chair experiment, it is possible to ask them to try saying "no" to the person they cannot say it to and then to carry out a dialogue by moving to the other person's place. Such people are greatly affected not only by what the people they like are saying but also by what those who they do not like and even do not know well might say. For example, confluent people are greatly distressed when someone says, "How selfish you are," even when it is not true. In such cases, experiments on refusing untrue statements can be carried out during therapy.

All these shows that the purpose of work carried out on confluence during therapy is the development of the self-support systems of the person and to have the client acknowledge his/her responsibilities. Self- support is the awareness of all internal and external resources and alternatives and the ability to use them (Clarkson and Mackewn 1993, 108). In order for a person to be self-supporting, he/she has to be fully aware of what is going on at the existing moment, to be able to make plans for the future, to be able to develop alternatives, and to have the strength to use the past as a creative resource.

One of the most important factors in self-support is physical processes (Joyce and Sills 2003, 84). When people are tired, hungry, or physically unwell, they find it difficult to support themselves. Hence, the first condition for people to gain the power for self-support is to be aware of their bodily needs and to meet them in a healthy manner. Another body-related subject that should be considered in terms of self- support is the way the body is used and breath is taken. For example, there is a vast difference in what a person feels when talking with shoulders hunched, bent from the waist and holding his/her breath, and what he/she feels while talking when comfortably seated in an armchair, shoulders opened up, and breathing regularly.

Another factor that is important in terms of self-support is the language a person uses. For example, if the person constantly holds others responsible for whatever happens ("You are making me very angry by acting like this"), renders himself helpless ("He has a grudge against me, what can I do?") or acts the victim ("Nobody has shown me any closeness so far"), it will not be possible for him/her to support him/herself. The self-supporting person starts his/her sentences with "I" rather than "you" or "he/she." For example, expressions such as "I get angry when you act like this," "I don't agree with you on this," or "I believe that the opinions I have stated are correct" help the person both in expressing him/herself clearly and in accepting the responsibility for his/her feelings, thoughts, and beliefs. In this way, the person can lay claim to his/her own strength. The person who is able to self- support identifies with what he/she is experiencing (Sills et al. 1998, 125). In other words, the self-supporting person, instead of avoiding situations that create stress and lead to negative feelings, tries to accept, understand, and solve them. In order to achieve this, once the person determines the situation, he/she has to make certain suggestions to him/herself about what could be done related to such a situation. For example, statements such as "He has a grudge against me and I will talk to him about this as soon as possible" or "Nobody shows me any closeness, and I will start with reviewing my behavior first in order to find out the causes of this" get the person out of the helpless and victim roles. Therefore, it is very important for the therapist to concentrate on changing the language the client uses and help him/her in gaining strength for self-support.

One other factor that is important in terms of self-support is the ability to use environmental resources. Having the power for self- support does not mean doing everything by oneself. The person who is able to self-support is aware of how, from whom, and when he/she can ask help (Joyce and Sills 2003, 84). For example, in order to support him/herself, a person can join a gymnasium, register to an art course, practice yoga or meditation, start playing a musical instrument, read to make up for his/her lack of knowledge on certain subjects, or attend conferences, take part in individual or group therapies, or even discover entirely different ways.

Developing one's self-support system by using environmental supports is the basis of the maturing process. However, using environmental resources does not mean manipulating the people in the environment. In other words, using environmental supports does not involve forcing others to behave in a certain way, to make them feel guilty by exploiting their feelings, to ask them to decide for us, or to take on our responsibilities. People with a tendency for confluence could also try to manipulate the therapist. As such people are afraid of making mistakes, making decisions by themselves, taking on responsibility and do not trust themselves, they always expect others to do something for them. When this is the case—when others are always taking responsibility for them, doing something for or instead of them—they can never mature and gain their self-confidence. They remain dependent on other people.

Consequently, one of the primary tasks of the therapist is to help the client to become aware of these manipulations.

When helping the client to become aware of his/her manipulations, the dialogue established between the therapist and the client is of utmost importance. The therapist, by supporting the client through the dialogic relationship, contributes to his/her gaining the strength for self-support. Perls (1973, 51) indicated that in supporting the client, to have the therapist listen to the client completely and with all his/her being, and to refrain from judgment is highly effective. Supporting the client does not mean giving advice, making decisions for the client or interpreting the client's actions for him/her. Once the therapist manages to make the client aware of his/her manipulations, he/she then disappoints the client by not showing the expected reactions to these manipulations. For example, some clients try to force the therapist with questions such as "Can you tell me what the right thing is for me to do about this?" "How do you think I should act in this situation?" "What should I say to him?" or "Should I leave her?" Some clients become angry when the therapist does not give the answers they are expecting and could start to accuse the therapist. For example, they may make accusations such as "You are not helping me at all," "I am not benefiting from the therapy," or "You are not fulfilling your obligations." In such cases, the therapist should explain the point of view of the Gestalt approach regarding these issues, should be understanding in the face of such questions and accusations, and should orient the client toward finding the answers to their questions by themselves. During this orientation, the therapist should never try to impose his/her value judgments and truths on the client, and via creative indifference, should work on his/her side and with him/her in order to enable the client to reach his/her own truths. In such manipulative situations, the therapist should be extremely sensitive, should neither prevent the development of the self-support strength of the client with ready answers, nor make him/her feel alone and helpless.

In conclusion, through confluence, awareness of boundaries is seriously impaired. Compared to other types of contact, confluence is the most insidious one (Korb et al. 1989, 60). Thus, it is not very easily detected. At the end of the work carried out on confluence during therapy, people become individuals who can own their desires, needs, and feelings, who can show respect to themselves and others for their differences, and who are free and self-supporting.

15

POLARITIES

Polarities are one of the most significant concepts in the Gestalt approach, and Jung's archetypes are at its root. According to Jung (1954/1968), archetypes are the structural components of the collective unconscious and have emotional elements. Characters from mythology, legends, sagas, folk stories, fairy tales, and history lie at the base of archetypes. Various characters such as God, the devil, woman, man, hero, angel, witch, king, queen, and persecutor are examples. Various characteristics of these archetypes are included in our personalities to a greater or lesser extent and cause polarizations. In Eastern philosophy, it is also believed that there are two different and opposing energies called yin and yang within the person.

Following Jung and Eastern philosophy, the Gestalt therapy approach states that people are born possessing both the characteristics of all archetypes and yin/yang energy. In this view, in order for a characteristic to emerge, its opposite also has to come out simultaneously (Clarkson and Mackewn 1993, 44). For example, in order to say that a person is happy, we must have observed that he/she is not sad, or in order to say that someone is polite, we must have observed that he/she was not rude. Hence, for one of these two opposing characteristics to become clear, the other must move to the background, and thus in a way, both characteristics are emerging simultaneously. In other words, happy and sad, polite and rude, considerate and inconsiderate, responsible and irresponsible, or calm and excitable are different extremes, different aspects of the same thing. Therefore, in the Gestalt approach, it is believed that each personality trait exists on a spectrum and at each end of this are characteristics that are opposites (Fantz 1998, 115). These personality traits can be shown linearly as follows:

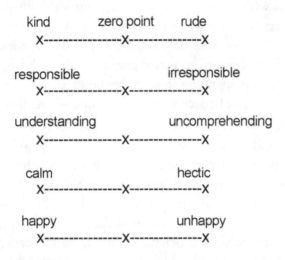

At the middle of two opposite personality traits on the same spectrum is a neutral place where the two poles are in balance (Perls 1947/1992, 9). This place, which is also called the zero point, is equidistant from both ends. As long as a person stays at the zero point, he/she will be equally distant from being polite or rude and thus can easily move toward one according to his/her needs and environmental conditions.

The Gestalt Perspective on Polarities

Evaluation of a Polarity as Good or Bad Is Determined According to the Person's Needs and Environmental Conditions

According to the Gestalt approach, it is not appropriate to evaluate a pole, that is, a personality trait, as either good or bad without taking into consideration the needs and environmental conditions of the person.

A personality trait such as being calm or excitable is actually neither a bad nor a good characteristic. The important thing is to decide when, to what extent, and toward whom to be calm or excitable by considering one's needs and environmental alternatives. For example, there is no doubt that when you are socializing, when you are with your friends or family, to be calm is beneficial—a good thing in terms of maintaining good relations with others. However, when you realize that a pickpocket is about to snatch your purse; to act calmly would not be good, because if you do not act fast, you may soon be left with no money. Similarly, while being clean seems to be a good characteristic both hygienically and socially, if you start spending four to five hours each day washing your hands or body, as can be seen in obsessive-compulsive disorders, then it will not be a good trait at all.

While standing at the zero point, in order to be able to decide to which pole and to what extent a person should go, the person has to know very well how to behave according to the poles located on that spectrum. In other words, the person should be able to choose to be industrious or lazy, to be stable or unstable, as the situation requires. If the person lacks the skill to behave according to the demands of both these poles, then he/she will fail to give the appropriate reactions and will be unable to make healthy contact.

For example, people who can establish healthy contacts do not have difficulty in saying "yes" or "no" to others depending on the situation. Hence, since they do not say "yes" to everything whether necessary or not, when they do say "yes," they really mean it and enjoy what they are doing; they do not feel angry about doing something because they reluctantly said "yes." On the other hand, those who say "no" to whatever comes destroy the possibility of sharing something and will be deprived of the pleasure of enjoying doing something for others.

Disowned Poles Lead to Inner Conflicts

According to the Gestalt approach, people are neither good nor bad when they are born. They learn not to show some of those characteristics seen as bad, wrong, or inappropriate by society, while exhibiting certain other traits depending on the value judgments of their environment. However, even if we do not want to accept those of our characteristics that are not approved of by society and if we try to hide them even from ourselves, they do not disappear but continue their existence like a shadow in our subconscious. For example, while people want to have character traits such as politeness, responsibility, and joy, which are seen by society as positive, they do not want to be rude, irresponsible, or sad, which the society regards as negative. These negative sides that remain in the shadows cannot develop and thus always have the potential to emerge in an exaggerated and primitive manner. This, in turn, leads people to be more afraid of their hidden sides and to reject them.

According to the Gestalt approach, the failure of a person to move along the various character spectra, to judge certain character traits as bad no matter what his or her needs and environmental conditions are, and always to show the same type of behavior is an unhealthy way of living. For example, if a person thinks that he/she should be strong at all times and in whatever conditions, he/she can never tolerate feeling weak. Even when necessary, he/she neither shares problems with others nor asks for help. This prevents him/her from establishing close relationships with others and eventually makes him/her lonely. Some people, on the other hand, do not get stuck at one of these poles but perpetually drift from one to the other without considering their needs and environmental conditions. They may be calm one day and angry on another in response to the same incident or love a person one day and hate him/her on another day. Whether stuck at a certain pole or drifting from one to the other, these people hate to be criticized and immediately become defensive. Since even the slightest possibility of having a characteristic that they regard as negative scares them greatly, they deny and project it onto others. They have rigid and stereotypical beliefs about themselves. As such people accept only one of the poles, they have a lot of characteristics that they are not aware of, as well as a number of blind spots. They experience inner conflict because of these blind spots, and this leads to the emergence of neurotic symptoms (Zinker 1997, 200).

Polarities can emerge on every issue and at any time because we are the ones who create them (Latner 1986, 99). Polarization can occur among hundreds of different characteristics such as feelings and logic, adequacy and inadequacy, stupidity and brightness, dependency and independency, maturity and immaturity, honesty and falsity. Polarization can also be experienced between our victim and executioner parts, witch and angel sides, or sinner and wise manners. Even though poles have great variety, the ones most focused on in the Gestalt approach are those of topdog and underdog. The dominant one is the topdog while the one less recognized is the underdog (Clarkson and Mackewn 1993, 105). Topdog corresponds to the superego of the psychoanalytic approach and is the part that gives orders to the person about what should be done. This part can be described as the person's critical, fault-finding, accusatory, demanding, and dictatorial side. Topdog is generally the irrational, rigid, and ruling side. It is always right, hard to satisfy and wants the underdog to live according to its standards. It perpetually creates pressure with commands such as "Be clean," "Be punctual," "Be responsible," and "Be industrious," which are in accord with societal value judgments. When these are not actualized, then it demeans the underdog with insults such as you are "stupid," "unreliable," "lacking will power," and "clumsy."

The underdog is passive and helpless. It finds the demands of the topdog justified and accepts its insults. While it responds on one hand with "Yes, you are right, I am not a good person," "I am bad, inadequate, selfish, and greedy," on the other, it responds with "Don't be mad at me," "Look, I am trying," "I forgot," or "I will do it first tomorrow," or other such explanations (Latner 1986, 122). While the topdog has mostly sadistic characteristics, the underdog is a masochist. According to Perls (1969, 85), despite the fact that the topdog is much more dominant and strong, the winner of the conflict is the underdog because by finding excuses, by avoiding, or procrastination, it sabotages the topdog and prevents it from acting. The underdog's being the winner of the conflict actually results in the failure of the person to achieve what he/she wants. What causes the inner conflict to emerge is the fact that the person expends his/her energy on hiding or ignoring those traits that he/she has but does not acknowledge. However, this is a futile effort because these unacknowledged and denied characteristics emerge sooner or later, and the conflict between the characteristics that the person finds positive and those regarded as negative arises. The dominant side fights with the rejected, hidden side (Clarkson and Mackewn 1993, 105). This fight between the opposite poles paralyses the person, renders him/her immobile, and leads to the person being stuck. Perls et al. (1951/1996, xiii) tried to explain this situation with this question: "If you had two helpers who were constantly fighting, how much work could you expect from them?" On the other hand, no matter how little the person is aware of his/her characteristics that he/she regarded as negative and tries to cover them up, they nevertheless emerge in the most unsuspected situations and in an unexpected manner. In other words, the more a person exaggerates one of the poles, after a while or under different circumstances, the other pole will emerge in just as exaggerated manner as the other. For example, a person who is very industrious can eventually become a person who cannot do any work at all, or a person who is generally very sensitive can become totally the opposite.

Such people believe that if they accept their negative sides, they will always act according to their negative sides. For example, a person who acknowledges his/her aggressive side is afraid of attacking constantly, a person who owns up to his/her selfish behavior is afraid of being selfish forever, or a person who accepts acting irresponsibly is afraid of being irresponsible always. However, once the person accepts such traits, he/she realizes that there is a choice to behave one way or the other. Thus they give themselves the freedom to be aggressive, selfish, or irresponsible when they feel it appropriate and act otherwise when necessary (Zinker 1997, 205). If the person becomes aware of these polarized characteristics and knows that they are located on a dimension and complement each other, then he/she can use his/her energy to move more easily between these poles and be more flexible rather than fighting with him/herself. Latner (1986, 122) indicated that, for the development of a balanced and integrated personality, the thesis and antithesis of the poles has to reach a synthesis. A person who owns all his/her poles, that is, a person who has achieved the integration of his/her poles is actually a very "wealthy" person. Since such a person has a wide-ranging and creative behavior repertoire, he/she can reach his/her goals under any conditions.

Would you like to write down the personality traits that you think you possess now? First, list those that occur to you immediately and then write their opposites next to them. Are there any traits among these that you think as negative, such as aggression, lying, gossiping, or indecision? If there are traits that you think are negative, try to figure out situations where these could be useful and even necessary. Imagine how much your life could change if you acknowledged these characteristics.

How to Work with Polarities in Therapy

The purpose of pole-related work during therapy is to enable the client

a. To become aware of those poles he/she is denying

b. To acknowledge them

c. To resolve the emerging inner conflict

d. To integrate the poles which are on the same dimension (Yontef 1993, 59)

During therapy, in order to integrate the poles, first they have to be completely separated from one another. To that end, it is very important to define the names and characteristics of the poles. Every person has his/her own poles, and each pole has its own name (Clarkson and Mackewn 1993, 107). Some poles (such as masculine/feminine, strong/weak, happy/unhappy) can be easily identified by the client. Some are less clear and be given different names depending on the phenomenology of the client (Joyce and Sills 2003, 136). For example, the opposite of being rigid could be being soft for someone, being unconventional for another, and being easygoing for somebody else. Hence, before starting pole-related work in therapy, sufficient time should be allotted to defining and naming both poles, and haste should be avoided. For example, one day Judith complained about her daughter being very demanding and always asking for things. When she said "no" to her daughter's demands, she not only felt bad but also sparked conflict with her daughter. When she said "yes," she still felt bad and, this time, an inner conflict started. While exploring what caused Judith to feel bad in both cases, it became apparent that when she did not meet the demands of her daughter, she saw herself as selfish and as a bad mother, and when she met her demands, she felt highly pressured and helpless. Upon this discovery, Judith first wanted to name her poles selfish and helpless. Then she realized that these were not wholly appropriate and changed the names to "bad mother" and "good mother." While talking about the definitions of the bad and good mother, she realized that these names were not appropriate either and finally named her poles "self-protecting" and "not self-protecting."

Once the names and characteristics of the poles have been defined, a dialogue can be requested between the two employing the two-chair technique. For example, to continue the above example, Judith talked as her self-protecting side when sitting in one chair and as her not self-protecting side while in the other. The purpose of setting up a dialogue between two poles in therapy is to make the client fully aware of the thoughts, feelings, and needs of both sides, as well as their expectations from each other. This awareness allows the person to change his/her point of view, to integrate these poles, and thus to resolve conflict. Greenberg (1979) showed that the two-chair technique is important in the following five respects:

1. To separate out both sides and to let them contact with each other
2. To help the client to take his/her own responsibility
3. To be aware of the factors that perpetuate the conflict
4. To clarify the conflict
5. To fully express the feelings and thoughts of both sides

Before starting the two-chair practice in therapy, the client is informed about how the dialogue is to be set up. In general, it may be more helpful to start the dialogue with the rejected or unaccepted pole because the client is less aware of what this side is thinking and what it is feeling. Because of this, the client could initially find it hard to start the dialogue from the disowned side. Hence, the therapist should help the client both to demonstrate how this experiment can be carried out and to make it easier for the client to recognize his/her disowned side. When deemed appropriate, the therapist can enlighten the client about the topdog and underdog. It is very important that during dialogue work the therapist should be in creative indifference (Perls 1969, 15), which means that the therapist will not be taking sides with one of the client's poles and will not orient the client toward his/her own opinions. More detailed information on this is given in the chapter on resistance. The task of the therapist is to help the client to fully express and be aware of both poles. In the end, it is the client who determines how he/she will achieve integration and what sort of decision he/she will reach. In some cases, during the dialogue between the poles, introjected information or unfinished business may emerge and cause the dialogue to be blocked.

In such situations, first the introjected messages have to be corrected so that the dialogue can continue. For example, Ruth, who had divorced three years previously and had a six-year-old son, realized that when a man was interested in her, she would cool her attitude toward him using projection and deflection in particular and finally would start to mistreat him. On the other hand, Ruth said that what she really wanted was to remarry. Under these circumstances, the remarriage of the client did not seem very likely because she was experiencing an inner conflict. While one side of her was feeling lonely and looking for a partner, the other side was sabotaging and blocking her. When she was asked to set up a dialogue between these two sides, she chose to name the poles topdog and underdog, the side which wanted to marry being the underdog. A part of the dialogue work carried out with this client is given below.

Underdog: *I am so lonely, how nice it would be to have a boyfriend. He would make my life easier.*

Topdog: *Make your life easier? He will only make it harder. You will have to take care of him too.*

Underdog: *Why should he make it harder? My life is not easy now anyway.*

Topdog: *You have a child. You must take care of him. What happens if they cannot get along? Maybe your son won't like him.*

Underdog: *Why shouldn't he like him if he is a nice person?*

Topdog: *You should be self-sufficient, all men are the same. They will hurt you sooner or later. You were so happy to get married, look what it came to. Won't you ever be smart?*

Underdog: *All right, most men could be like that, but . . .*

Topdog: *Not most of them, all of them. Your father is the same; He doesn't get along with your mother. They didn't divorce, but you know how many times you thought, "I wish they would divorce." Just don't rock the boat.*

Underdog:	*That may be true but not all of them. I can't like anybody because of you anyway. You find something wrong with everybody. His look, his family, you even disgraced someone in my eyes just because he did not pronounce a word correctly. He is actually a very nice person.*
Topdog:	*There you go, all of them have some faults. Don't ask for trouble, sit tight. Just be with your child and take care of him. He is more important than you. He could be unhappy; do you want him to be unhappy?*
Underdog:	*Will he be unhappy* (she starts to tear up, and her voice becomes lower). Of *course I don't want him to be unhappy.*
Topdog:	*Sure, he will be unhappy. And he will be sharing you with someone else. He is what is important. You have no right to make him unhappy.*
Underdog:	*Yes, you are right, I guess* (she started to cry quietly).

As can be seen, even though it seems as if the topdog has convinced the underdog, the fact that Ruth is crying at the end of the dialogue indicates that their conflict is not wholly resolved. The most important argument the topdog raises against the underdog's wish to marry is Ruth's son. Here it could be said that Ruth's beliefs related with motherhood, which has been introjected but not assimilated, lies at the base of her conflict. While working with the introjected message, Ruth talked about how both her mother and father thought that children were more important than anything else, how they agreed that the most important and even the only obligation of a woman was to take care of her children and to be a good mother, how her parents disagreed on many issues but definitely shared the same opinion on this, and how her mother stopped working after having children even though she loved working very much. Hence it became clear that the message Ruth had introjected regarding motherhood was that "mothers should give up all their desires for their children." After Ruth was helped in returning this introjected message to her parents and in defining the correct message for her, the dialogue between the topdog and underdog was once more taken up.

The final goal of working with polarities is the resolution of conflict and the achievement of integration (Fantz 1998, 115). In order to achieve integration, it is not sufficient merely to have both sides listening to each other; there also has to be mutual acceptance. For example, Frank started his work on polarities with expressions such as "You don't deserve to live, you are a bad person, your life is bad" and "You have no good side." Frank had difficulty in accepting this side of him that was very rigid, extremely cruel, and accusatory. He was always trying to silence it and not to listen to it, but he could not save himself from its influence. During the session, he talked in tears about how, when he was about seven or eight years old, the children in his neighborhood used to make fun of him because of his being jug-eared and how they often beat him. While telling about his memories, he realized that although on one hand he was very angry with those children, on the other hand he also identified with them and was self-critical just like them, making fun of himself; that is, he became his own enemy. This awareness enabled him to view his critical, cruel, and accusatory side with a greater tolerance. Now, when he was acting in a hostile manner toward himself, instead of trying not to hear this side, he was able to say, "I know you suffered a lot, you are my teased and beaten side. I feel sorry for you. I am really sorry that you had to shoulder this task, but you no longer need to criticize me. You know that I am a good person." After a while, Frank heard this side very seldom, and he considerably reduced his rigid and cruel behavior against himself.

Different techniques can be used during work on integration of polarities. One of these is to ask the client to talk about or act as one of his/her poles by exaggerating it. For example, if one of the poles is "controller," the person could be asked to express and exaggerate his /her controller side by trying to control everything in the room. Another way is to make the clients draw their poles. To make a mask of the disowned side is another way that can be used.

According to Latner (1986, 55), integration of poles is an "aha" type experience. An "aha" experience is a discovery, and through it, clients change themselves as well as the structure of their environment. They reorganize their environment by starting to think and act differently. This is not just an intellectual change but a total transformation of the person. Now, the former conflict has changed places with a new behavior, a new "I," a new world. This new Gestalt formed as a result of the "aha" experience, like a pebble thrown in a pool, first spreads out in ripples and then slowly calms down. Thus it no longer catches our attention because it has become a part of us. A victory is won through integration, but in this victory, there is no defeated or victimized side; both sides are winners.

In summary, the Gestalt approach presents a wealth of effective ways that can be applied in the resolution of inner conflicts. However, in order to be able to apply these techniques, the therapist must have integrated the Gestalt theory and methods within him/herself. Otherwise, it is possible to cause the disintegration rather than the integration of the client. In therapy, starting to work on polarities should not be attempted before the client has achieved a sufficient level of self- support power. Furthermore, the client should never be rushed or forced into integration. In particular, work on polarities should be avoided in border case personality disturbances and psychotic cases.

PART III:
APPLICATION

16

RESISTANCE

In its most general sense, resistance is knowing what must be done but being unable to do it. For example, if you are watching television instead of studying or going on a diet every Monday but coming off every Tuesday, then you are resisting the academic success or weight loss. If you are habitually late to wherever you should go, if you forget what you were supposed to do, or if you are constantly procrastinating, then it again means that you are resisting something. Although as a child you were told to sit up straight by your parents and teachers to repeatedly, the failure to make this posture habitual also indicates resistance. In order to be resistant, the person has to have a specific goal such as visiting a friend, reading an article, or preparing a meal. Every personal obstruction that prevents the realization of these goals is resistance. To reach the goals, the obstructions have to be eliminated.

Resisting something, that is to one's benefit or avoiding doing something while knowing that it should be done actually, means harming oneself. For example, buying expensive things despite the truth that you will go broke or not doing your chores knowing that you will be scolded for it are undoubtedly against your benefit. According to Karon (1976, 203), there are three possible reasons for self-harming behavior. The first is having a "weak will." The basic belief of this point of view is that a person can change if he/she really wants to. If the person is not able to change, then it means that he/she either does not want to change or does not put in sufficient effort. The other possible reason for a person's harmful behavior is being "irrational." The basic belief of this point of view is that a rational person would definitely want to change these self- harming behaviors. The third possible reason is the inability to give up habits. The basic belief of this point of view is that a person who is sufficiently insistent and keeps on trying can get rid of his/her bad habits and adopt new ones. If these point of views are valid, then how can we explain the situations where a person both wants to and makes an effort to change but cannot change? Why do clients, despite coming to therapy to be free of their complaints, and despite making a great effort and spending considerable time, still continue to harm themselves and resist change? Various psychotherapy approaches, seeking an answer to these questions, claimed that resistance is a much more complicated concept and could not be understood via the above explanations, and so they leaned toward others.

Even though different therapy approaches have put forward different explanations and focused on different points regarding resistance, they have all refrained from judging a person for showing resistance, as in the aforementioned explanations, and on the contrary, have tried to investigate the meaning and the function of resistance for that particular person. While doing this, the most significant point of view put forth and accepted by various therapy approaches is the fact that resistance protects the person against something, which is to say that it helps the person to defend him/herself. For example, while Freud (1938/1966) defines resistance as "a defense developed against inner impulses that threaten the personality of a person," Reich (1945/1972), another pioneer of the psychoanalytic approach and who influenced the Gestalt approach, describes resistance as "a bodily defense against unacceptable memories." Additionally, both have indicated that resistance should be "overcome" during therapy.

The Gestalt Approach Viewpoint on Resistance

Regarding resistance as a defense is also one of the fundamental viewpoints of the Gestalt approach. In the beginning, the Gestalt approach was influenced very much by the psychoanalytic approach, and even the "interruptions to contact" were labeled as "resistances to contact" in those days because of this psychoanalytic legacy (Clarkson 1991, 91). Despite these influences, however, there are significant differences between the Gestalt approach and psychoanalysis in terms of how resistance is approached in therapy.

Perls first mentioned the Gestalt perspective on resistance in 1936 in a paper titled "Oral Resistances" presented to the International Psychoanalysis Conference that was convened in Czechoslovakia (referred to in Clarkson and Mackewn 1993, 14–15). In this paper, he tried to explain the concept through the resistance of a baby to the mother's milk. There is no doubt that mother's milk is essential for a child's growth. However, no matter how useful and beneficial it is, if the baby is not hungry, has colic, is sleepy, or if another of his/her needs is more dominant, then the baby will not suckle and, despite all of the mother's efforts, will show resistance. In a similar way, at the bottom of a person's failure to behave in a way that appears to be useful and even necessary, might lie other needs that cannot be clearly observed from the outside.

According to the Gestalt viewpoint, resistance occurs when we try to impose our "rights" onto others. In other words, resistance is a person's self-defense and protection, preserving his/her integrity and survival against externally imposed pressure (Zinker 1994, 118). The person is protecting him/herself from perceived harm by showing resistance. The instinct to protect oneself is one of the innate characteristics of a person, and thus it cannot be eradicated. If attempts are made to destroy this instinct, then the person moves away from his/her natural drives and cannot sustain his/her psychological integrity and balance (Kepner 1987, 61). Hence, self-protection is the most natural right of a person. Who can give up self-protection because somebody tells him/her that there is no danger? Who can be asked to give up his/her right to protect his/her integrity even if it is for his/her own good?

For these reasons, in Gestalt therapy, resistance is not a situation to be eliminated but something to be understood, explored, and experienced. Resistance is a part of the person. This means that both the one who wants to change and the one who shows resistance is the person him/herself. Hence, breaking down or eliminating resistance during therapy means breaking down and eliminating a capacity of the self (Kepner 1987, 65). A therapist who regards resistance as something to be broken down or eliminated is actually being disrespectful to the client's right to self-defense. Without understanding the meaning of resistance, the reasons behind its emergence, from what and how it protects the person, what are the needs that underlie it, and without carrying on work related to these, elimination of resistance could lead to a short-term change, but the generalization and effectiveness of that change will be low in the long term.

The dialectical opposite of the word resistance is "assistance" (Clarkson and Mackewn 1993, 115). This means that resistance and assistance are two poles of the same continuum. Perls et al. (1951/1996, 276) suggested several times that "resistance" could be renamed assistance but later changed their minds; however, they remained insistent that in order to make it clear that resistance is used in a different sense than it had been in the psychoanalytic approach, it should always be placed in quotation marks (referred to in Clarkson and Mackewn 1993, 115). However, for practical reasons, the word resistance is not placed in quotation marks in contemporary publications related with the Gestalt therapy approach.

According to the Gestalt approach, it is believed that resistance has its origins in the "creative adjustment" made in the past.

Creative Adjustment

Humans are born with the innate capacity to be aware of their needs and the demands of the environment, and they are innately equipped with everything necessary to choose from the available opportunities that are beneficial for themselves (Crocker 1999, 19). A person's ability to harmonize his/her needs and wishes with the environmental conditions for his/her own benefit becomes possible through "creative adjustment" (Yontef 1993, 195). A person who adjusts creatively is aware of both his/her needs and wishes and the environmental factors, and in order to adapt these two, creates various ways and produces alternatives. In an adjustment that is not creative, the person behaves according to the standards determined by the environment without taking his/her needs into consideration. On the other hand, to have creativity where there is no adjustment leads to various hardships and causes the person to feel alone or empty. There is no standard formula for creative adjustment (Latner 1992, 27): it is unique to the individual. It is determined by each person him/herself according his/her needs and environmental factors. Therefore, the solutions that a person will find through creative adjustment and eventually what he/she will achieve cannot be known beforehand. The person tries to create the best adjustment for him/herself under the existing conditions, but this adjustment still might not be the best solution when the conditions change. For example, for a child who is frequently verbally or physically abused by his parents, to stay away from his parents can be seen as a good creative adjustment, but keeping a distance in adulthood from everybody with no distinction is not a good solution. However, what should be remembered regarding creative adjustment is the fact that no matter what a person is doing, it is the best he/she can do under the existing conditions (Latner 1992, 28). Creative adjustment is an indicator that shows how the person has dealt with the physical and psychological threats under which they previously lived (Mackewn 1999, 170). When born, a baby needs other people to satisfy his/her needs. When hungry, soiled, in pain, or sleepy, the baby conveys this to others by crying and expects his/her needs to be met. When he/she becomes a little older, his/her needs vary more and grow richer. For instance, needs such as love, attention, and appreciation start to emerge. In order to meet these needs, the child starts to behave according to his/her environment that is according to what his/her parents and others are offering him/her and also according to their rules, as otherwise he/she cannot get what he/she wants. For example, a child who is scolded by his/her parents when making noise or objecting, can, in time, make a creative adjustment and learn to be quiet and not to express his/her needs so forcefully. Similarly, a child who loves action and jumping around gets a negative reaction from his/her parents and is not allowed to play in the garden either might eventually, through creative adjustment, start not to move around much and might become reluctant even to stand up. Different children might choose different ways of adjustment even when they live under the same conditions. The best examples of this are from siblings. Despite the fact that they live in the same home and hence face the same reactions, siblings generally have different personalities. For example, in a home where the children are never allowed to cry and where crying is considered to be very irritating, through creative adjustment, in order not to cry, one child might develop a pattern of acting roughly and with cruelty, another one might develop a pattern of being very sensitive to the needs of others, yet another might develop a pattern of contacting in a very cold manner, and the youngest might develop a pattern of whining constantly.

Most of the clients come to therapy for problems arising from behavior patterns that were once indicators of creative adjustment but later turned into fixed Gestalts. For example, the reason Kate came for therapy was the problems she had in her relationship with her boyfriend. When Kate was a little girl, like all children she needed her father's attention and love. Every evening, when the doorbell rang, she rushed to welcome her father before anybody else. Once the father was inside, he would hold her, tell her nice things, and sometimes even bring her little presents. However, after ten minutes or so, her father's interest decreased, and he would want to do other things, such as having dinner, watching television, or engaging in other activities. Hence, after ten minutes, he dismissed Kate, by saying, "Go and play with your toys," "Do your homework," or "It is bedtime." If Kate ignored these instructions, continued sitting on his lap or did not leave him alone, then he would start getting tense and start scolding her. A few times when Kate refused to get down from his lap, this even went as far as his slapping her. As these situations became repetitive, Kate learned that she could not have her father's affection and attention for more than ten minutes, and with a creative adjustment, she started to go to her room and to get away from him before he even said anything. In this way, Kate protected herself from being scolded by her father and from losing his love, and also she could have the affection and attention she craved, even if only for a short while. Even though she could not get plenty of the attention and love she needed, this was the best solution she could find under these circumstances. In her thirties, Kate, realizing that she still could not manage to have a happy relationship with a man, applied for therapy. During the therapy process, Kate became aware that she was also using the "get away after ten minutes" style with her boyfriends, that had been useful for her in her relations with her father. In her relationships, she chose either men who would not be interested in her for more than "ten minutes" or those who showed as much attention and love as she wanted, but as she herself did not know what to do after "ten minutes," she either picked a fight, sulked, or went into fits of jealousy. In the end, unsatisfied with the relationship, Kate broke up with them, or they left her because of the fights she started and her sulks. Kate reacted to her partners not according to their characteristics and the existing conditions but according to past conditions and the characteristics of her father. It was as if Kate was living in the past.

As can be seen in the example above, people who cannot form a healthy relationship and who behave according to the creative adjustment they made in the past are not aware of how they are behaving. Clients frequently express this as "I don't know what I am doing that spoils my relationships." Since they are not aware of what they are doing, they cannot decide about what to change. Instead, they perpetuate the same behavior patterns that made them feel safe and protected in the past. Even if friends or relatives suggest different ways, since they do not know how to behave differently, they disregard these suggestions. On the other hand, as they are not experienced in different modes of behavior and as they have no idea what they will face if they behave differently, they are scared to take such a path. Hence, they go on behaving as they have been used to and, in the end, find themselves stuck. They cannot reach out to new experiences and cannot develop themselves. Actually what should be done is to develop new creative adjustments appropriate for the changing environmental conditions, but the person is resisting to change.

During therapy, the resistance arising from past creative adjustments is approached according to the paradoxical theory of change. Resistance leads to impasses, and the therapist works with the impasse through creative indifference. Before going into possible interventions that can be used in therapy to deal with resistance, it will be useful to review in detail the concepts of the paradoxical theory of change, impasse, and creative indifference.

Paradoxical Theory of Change

As in all psychotherapy approaches, the goal of the Gestalt therapy approach is to help the client to change and develop. However, the Gestalt perspective on change is vastly different from that of the others as it is based on the paradoxical theory of change. According to this theory, change is not achieved by trying to be somebody that one isactually not; on the contrary, it comes about through trying to be one's true self.

In order to understand the paradoxical theory of change, the example of a plane flying in a certain direction can be used. If you look at a plane from very far away and for a very short time, then it seems to be standing still at a certain point and not moving. However, despite this perception the plane is actually traveling at a very high speed. Life consists of very short time segments following each other. The paradox here is splitting life into short time segments because time can never be stopped. In other words, even if at a certain moment the plane is perceived as merely hanging up in the air, both the plane and time are actually moving forward. Similarly, during therapy even if the client seems not to be changing at a certain moment, this does not indicate that he/she is not really changing. In other words, even if the person feels that he/she is not changing within a certain time segment, in reality, he/she is changing. Beisser (1970, 77), who developed the paradoxical theory of change, has encapsulated this as "change can only be possible by not changing within a given time segment." Wheeler and Backman (1994, 363) have stated regarding this paradoxical nature of change that during therapy, change cannot be actualized by forcing him/her to change either by the person him/herself or by someone else, but can only be achieved by expending efforts and time to be as he/she is.

As mentioned above, in traditional approaches, it is believed that change can be actualized through willpower, perseverance, and logic. In these approaches, the person is expected to change according to the "shoulds" imposed by the society. In contrast, according to the paradoxical theory of change, the harder a person is forced to change, the stronger will be the resistance to change. The human being, born with a basic driving force for growth and development, when provided with sufficient choices and when the conditions are convenient, will spontaneously choose the direction of growth and well-being and not need to resist (Clarkson 1991, 91).

Perls, who believed that nothing could be overcome with resistance, stated that the best way to overcome something is to go deeper into it (referred to in Naranjo 1993, 138). For example, if you are stubborn, exaggerate it, become even more stubborn. If you want to be spiteful, be more spiteful. When you really go deeply enough into it, you will see that at the end your stubbornness and spitefulness have disappeared, and they will have been assimilated. This principle lies in the basis of the Eastern martial arts Tai Chi Chuan and Judo. In these martial arts, the fighter defeats the opponents without opposing them but by deflecting their force back to them or pulling them further along in the direction of their movements. Just like the fighter who doesn't try to neutralize the opponent's force but instead uses it to beat him/her; the Gestalt therapist also does not try to eliminate resistance but uses its force.

Clients generally come to therapy with a predetermined notion of how they should be. They start therapy not only with a desire to leave behind them the feelings, thoughts, and behaviors that they do not like but also with a belief that they will change within a certain plan. Perls (1969, 37) also points this out and states that what most of the clients are expecting from therapy is not to actualize themselves but to actualize their self-image. Those clients who come to therapy to actualize their self-images want the therapist to take a side and to cooperate with the side that wants to change. Many therapists have reported achieving positive results by cooperating with the side of the client who wants to change. In contrast, in the Gestalt approach, it is believed that cooperating only with the change-desiring side of the client and ignoring the side that does not want to change will strengthen the inner conflicts of the client, and whatever success is achieved will not be long-term. Ignoring the side of the client that does not want to change and the failure to integrate it within the personality will lead to perpetuation of resistance in a covert way. This, in turn, causes lack of spontaneity, zest for life, or enthusiasm; it may even lead to the emergence of various illnesses or finally depression (Mackewn 1999, 65). Furthermore, to have the therapist cooperate only with the side that wants to change as the client expects also run contrary to the holistic perspective of the Gestalt approach.

According to Yontef (1993, 27), when a therapist tries to "lead" or "heal" the client, then the therapist is actually pushing or pressuring the client to be someone different, and this will result in increased resistance. In the end, the client not only shows resistance to his/her own processes but starts to resist the therapy and the therapist. Furthermore, the therapist who forces the client to change will also be insinuating messages such as "You are not adequate as you are," "I do not like you as you are," or "I can't accept you like this." These types of message cause the client to feel guilty and ashamed and to reinforce the negative feelings about him/herself. Hence, no matter how good the intentions are, forcing the client to change and trying to accelerate the change only serves the satisfaction of the therapist's need "to feel like a good therapist" but does no good for the client. If the therapist is disappointed with client's rate of change, then the actual reason is not the client but the therapist's own needs. In such a situation, the therapist should try to find out why he/she needs the client to change quickly and, if needed, should receive supervision. There is no doubt that to see the changes in the client is exciting for a therapist and makes him/her happy. However, forcing the client into rapid change will not engender "real" change. The purpose of therapy is not to push aside what the client is experiencing at that moment and fix something quickly (Crocker 1999, 228). The therapist, by pushing or hurrying, might enable the client to become aware of something or do something, but as long as the client's capacity for self-support is not developed, the generalization of the achieved results will be very low. Pushing and hurrying is particularly dangerous where hard-changing clients are concerned and can lead to serious problems in therapist-client relationships.

While reading the lines above, you might be asking yourself, "This is all very well, but if we do not push and hurry the client, how are we going to help those clients who are stuck at a certain point and who are even becoming worse?" According to the Gestalt approach, the answer to this question is hidden in the question itself. That is, the reason the client is getting worse is the fact that he/she is being forced and rushed to change. The clients' most important need is to feel that, even if they are not changing and remaining as they are, there is still a place for them in this world and they will not be rejected by the therapist because of their way of existence. A client who is rushed and forced to change cannot feel safe and accepted by the therapist. According to the Gestalt approach, as long as the client is not feeling safe and accepted, then he/she will not dare to put him/herself forth sincerely and as he/she is. The client will be tense and vigilant. Due to the effect of his/her instinct for self-protection, the client's contact with both him/herself and the therapist eventually starts to be interrupted and his/her resistance increases. How are you behaving on occasions where you do not feel safe and accepted? Can you fully establish contact with your environment? In a situation where contact is decreasing and resistance is increasing, the therapist should not push or rush the client to change but should on the contrary allow him/her to resist within a dialogic relationship and help him/her to experience his/her resistance to the full. In this way, the therapist enables the client to be aware of his/her two sides, the resisting side and wanting-to-change side. In the Gestalt approach, the situation where both the resisting and wanting-to-change sides appear concurrently is called an impasse.

Impasse

The concept of impasse is another innovation that the Gestalt approach has brought to the field of psychotherapy. At the point of impasse, the forces that want to grow and those that resist are engaged in a struggle (Clarkson and Mackewn 1993, 117). On one side of the impasse, there is the desire for growth, expansion, and change, while on the other side there is resistance, which is just as strong and is a result of behavior patterns born from creative adjustments established in the past (Joyce and Sills 2003, 131). The person experiencing an impasse is caught right in the middle and can move neither toward the side that wants to change nor to that which is resisting. The person is stuck and cannot act. Lubbock (1996) explains the impasse via the following scheme (referred to in Mackewn 1999, 172).

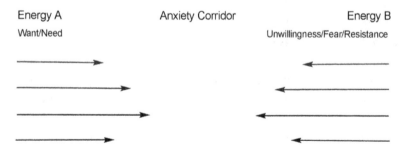

An impasse fosters catastrophic expectations of the unknown (Korb et al. 1989, 127). The person wants to change but is also afraid of this change because change means uncertainty, novelty, and lack of clarity. What is known and familiar always makes us feel safer. The person, even if not particularly satisfied with it, is used to his/her environment, knows what he/she can do, and what may happen. On the other hand, he/she does not know what is to come if changes occur, how to cope with them, and how to behave in the altered situation. For certain individuals, seeing new places, meeting new people, trying new food, or even dressing differently from the style he/she is used to can cause anxiety and fear. Furthermore, the person is not sure that the outcome of this change will be good. There is the risk of not liking the new places seen, disliking the new people, not enjoying the new food, or not feeling good in the new clothing style. The person cannot decide if it is worth taking such risks and also there is the risk of losing what one has through changing. All this paralyses the person; he/she is very confused, does not know what to do, and is consequently extremely anxious. The person in an impasse experiences an existential helplessness, is scared of being lost, and of finding him/herself in a void. The person in an existential impasse believes that he/she has no environmental support and no self-strength (Baumgardner and Perls 1975, 13).

In general, while clients and other psychotherapy approaches see the impasse as a negative situation, in the Gestalt approach, the impasse is seen as the zenith of potential for change resulting from a creative tension. According to Perls (1969, 76), the impasse is the most crucial point in therapy and is also the basis of growth. Every impasse is both a withdrawal from what is known and an approach to the unknown with slow and cautious steps. In order to be able to resolve the impasse, it is desirable for the client to experience it fully in therapy. To this end, the client is encouraged to feel as stuck, confused, empty, and helpless as much as possible, and in the meanwhile, he/she is helped to become aware of his/her feelings, thoughts and body. Fully experiencing the impasse during therapy is important for all clients, but this is especially so for those who show a tendency to resolve their impasse in an impulsive way or for those who expect the solution from the therapist. When, during therapy, the client becomes aware of the impasse with all its dimensions, his/her inner energy accelerates so rapidly that it becomes impossible to keep it in, and so it starts to come out. This is the point where the impasse starts unraveling.

In order to resolve an impasse during therapy, the covert conflicts underneath it have to be dealt with. One way of doing this could be to ask the client to create a dialogue between the two opposing sides. During this dialogue, in order to enable the client to realize the needs and value judgments of both sides of his/her impasse, he/she is invited to experience both sides bodily, emotionally, and cognitively. The therapist should act with creative indifference during the dialogue between the opposing sides.

Creative Indifference

The concept of creative indifference has roots in Zen Buddhism. According to Zen Buddhism the first condition of growing spiritually is "to accept" what "exists" as it is without being under the influence of any feelings or thoughts. Similarly, in the Gestalt approach, it is essential to accept the client and what goes on during therapy as they are.

In 1918, the philosopher Friedlander was the first to use the term *creative indifference* (referred to in Sills et al. 1998, 38). It is the middle point between two poles that are open to all possibilities or experiences coming from the environment without any prejudices or investments. The therapist who acts with creative indifference while displaying warm and sincere attention to the client during therapy also refrains from guiding the client toward a target that the therapist him/herself has defined. The therapist does not impose what he/she believes to be right on the client and does not force the client in a certain direction. Just like a gardener who, after providing the soil, seeds, air, and water necessary for the growth of a flower, and preventing the possible adverse environmental conditions, does not try to determine its color, smell, shape, or height while waiting for its growth, the therapist also having provided the necessary conditions for the growth of the client, does not preplan how, in which direction, or at what speed he/she will grow. In other words, creative indifference is the base that is required for the client to actualize him/herself. When the therapist prepares this base, then he/she trusts the client's process, believes that the client will choose what is best for him/herself, and respects his/her decisions. Through creative indifference, the therapist accepts not only the "good" or "correct" solutions of the client but his/her entire being as it is (Mackewn 1999, 174). Creative indifference gives the therapist the opportunity to see every characteristic of the client, the situation he/she is in, and both sides of the impasse he/she is experiencing (Perls et al. 19951/1996, 15). In this way, the therapist helps clients to recognize the disowned sides or characteristics in themselves or in the environment.

How to Work with Resistance in Therapy

The purpose of resistance work in the Gestalt approach is to make the client aware of his/her resistances and to take responsibility for them. Thus, resistance is seen as a very important tool in understanding and developing the personality, and for that reason, during therapy, the work is carried out not against but with resistance (Fantz 1998, 117). The task of the therapist is to help the client to name his/her resistances, to be aware of the underlying needs of such resistances, to own these needs, and to satisfy them by taking risks. During therapy, the answers to following questions are explored:

What is the client resisting?

How is the client resisting?

How is the client protecting him/herself?

Against what is the client protecting him/herself?

It is worth noting that the question, "Why is the client resisting?" is not included among the above questions, because "why" is a question that is not asked in the Gestalt approach (Perls 1973, 120). There are two important reasons for this. First, this question itself leads to resistance. For example, being asked "Why are you treating him like that?" will cause a feeling of being judged in many people and therefore will immediately lead to a defensive stand. The second reason for avoiding the "why" question is the fact that the answer given to this question in no way contributes to the solution to the problem.

The reasoning behind asking the "why" question is the belief that if we know the reasons for the problem, then we can solve it. According to this belief, in order to find a solution, the causes should be sought or, in other words, the solution is in the past. However, knowing the cause can never solve the psychological problem because (a) the roots of psychological problems generally lie in the childhood and most people do not accurately remember that period, (b) it is not possible to change the past, and (c) psychological problems almost never have a single cause. Let us assume that a person answers the question, "Why are you treating him like this?" with "Because I was brought up by my aunt and she was a very bad tempered person." In this case, since we cannot change what the person experienced in the past, then there is nothing we can do to solve the problem. Another reason for our inability to solve the problem in this way is that with such a response the person is putting the responsibility for his/her behavior onto somebody else, in this case, the aunt. For these reasons, in the Gestalt approach, instead of "why", "what" and "how" questions are used. For example, answers given to questions such as "What causes you to mistreat him?" "When do you mistreat him?" "How do you mistreat him?" and "How do you tell him what you want?" can lead us to the solution. The reasoning behind asking "what" and "how" questions are the belief that if we know the structure of the problem, then we can solve it (Perls 1969, 64). Hence, taking this belief as a starting point, in the Gestalt approach, the solution is sought in the structure of the problem that is in the present time as well as in the person experiencing the problem.

During therapy, there are many ways that can be used to investigate the structure of the problem. Perls et al. (1951/1996) claimed that all the experiments used in the Gestalt therapy approach are actually designed to raise awareness of resistances. What should be particularly remembered while working with resistance during therapy is that the client should be allowed to resist. Each client has a style of resistance that is unique. The therapist should be sensitive to the client's way of resisting and should support the client in experiencing resistance with awareness. During therapy, resistance can manifest itself in many ways, both overt and covert. For example, clients who speak nonstop during the therapy and giving the therapist no chance to talk, who have difficulty in finding examples, who keep silent for long periods, who come to the sessions late, who cancel sessions without notice or at the last minute, who despite saying how helpful the therapy is carry on self-damaging behaviors, who continuously ask the therapist for suggestions, or who do not want to carry out the proposed experiments, might be showing symptoms of covert resistance. Sometimes resistance might show itself through statements such as "I cannot concentrate today; I don't know where my mind is wandering." In such a case, the therapist can guide the client by saying, "Okay. Then don't try to concentrate, do the opposite and let your mind wander more." Or, if the client frequently answers the therapist's questions with "I don't know," then the therapist might ask him/her to exaggerate this situation by saying, "Keep on not knowing, even forget everything you know, and behave as if you know nothing." These are paradoxical interventions. The therapist has to be very careful while using them and explain why this experiment is suggested. Otherwise, if an explanation is not given, such interventions may cause feelings of guilt or shame in the client. Resistance sometimes appears with bodily or nonverbal reactions. In particular, the inconsistency between what the client is saying and his/her tone of voice, gestures and facial expressions, posture or breathing, could be indicators of resistance. It should also be kept in mind that some physical symptoms such as spasm, tension, pain, ache, burning sensation, and the like might also be related to resistance. How to work with the bodily resistances in therapy is discussed in detail in the body language section.

One other method that could be utilized while working with resistance in therapy is to ask the client to establish a dialogue between him/herself and his/her resistance. In such an experiment, first the client is required to liken his resistance to a wall and then to picture this wall in front of his/her eyes and describe it. Later, it is suggested that the client talk about him/herself as the wall. This experiment helps the client to be aware of to what he/she is resisting, to accept the resistance as a part of him/herself and also to take responsibility for his/her resistance. In one such experiment, Jane described the wall that is her resistance as this: I am a very high and wide brick wall. My color is mostly white, and I am rather damaged in some places. Where I am damaged, my paint has gone, in some places even the bricks are seen, and some of the bricks are broken. Later the dialogue between Jane and the wall continued as follows:

Jane: You look very high and very wide. I can't possibly get over you. When I face you, I feel helpless and small.

The Wall: Yes, I am high and wide. I feel so good. You can't possibly get over me. I am going to stay right here.

Jane: Why are you staying there? Why are you preventing me from getting over?

The Wall: I am staying here because I don't want you to do anything dangerous. If I didn't stand here and prevent you, then you would do something wrong and get into trouble. Because of me, you don't say "no" to people, you do what they want, and so they like you.

Jane: Yes, that is right. I want them to like me; I don't want to hurt anybody. But they say "no" to me, they hurt me. You can't protect me then.

The Wall: I can't prevent them from hurting you. I can only prevent you from hurting them. But nevertheless they like you.

Jane: If they liked me, they wouldn't hurt me. This has nothing to do with liking; they like me because I don't cause any trouble. If I do, then they don't like me. Actually they like my not causing any trouble. Nobody asks me what I think or what I want anyway.

The Wall: See! Well, actually you don't have any important ideas anyway. You don't know what you want either. You keep saying, "It makes no difference." Thanks to me, you don't bother to have any ideas. You don't waste time thinking about what you want. What else do you want?

Jane: Yes, most of the time, I don't know what I want, but sometimes I do. Also, even if not on everything, I still have certain ideas about some things and I want to express them.

The Wall: Hah! Say them aloud and make everyone laugh at you. How do you know those ideas are the right ones? And who cares about what you want?

Jane: I don't know. I wish they were important. Well, at least they are important for me. And why it is always somebody else's *ideas that are important? If you weren't there maybe I would talk more. Yes, you don't even look very strong. Wouldn't it be better to help me instead of obstructing me?*

The Wall: *I don't know if I can trust you. I am afraid of your becoming unhappy. No, I will not do it. I can't trust you.*

Jane's dialogue with the wall continued for a long time. However, as can be seen in the section given above, Jane started to recognize her fears related to not being liked and not being appreciated and also how the wall was trying to protect her. Toward the end of the dialogue, she started to stand up to it and even realize that it is not very strong.

While working with resistance in therapy, another experiment could be the establishment of a dialogue between the two sides causing the impasse. Such practices can play a significant role in the clarification of existential anxieties lying at the base of the impasse. Part of such a work carried out with Ruth is given below. When Ruth came for therapy, she was in an impasse in her relationship with her boyfriend. She neither wanted to leave him nor to change her behavior. During the previous sessions, Ruth had started to see how her desire to dominate her boyfriend and her jealousy were destroying their relation. However, Ruth was not aware of her other side, that is, the side that did not want to dominate and was not jealous. Her lack of awareness was playing a great role in the impasse. Being unaware of this side, Ruth always behaved in the same way and could not escape from the same vicious cycle. Hence, she was asked to create a dialogue between her two sides and she named them as "jealous and impassive."

Jealous: *I don't know you. How can you be so impassive? Your lover is about to walk away. He will cheat you and you will be alone, but you don't care.*

Impassive: *I don't understand you either. Actually he is going to run away because of you. Nag, nag, nag, you are always nagging him. "Why did you look in that direction? Why you said " hello" to her? Who is she? Why did you laugh at her? .*

Why you didn't laugh at her?" You are always asking never-ending questions. You are unbelievable. I feel stifled; your behavior makes me not only angry but also ashamed of you

Jealous: *I am also angry with you. How can you be so impassive? I am mad at you and I am also mad at all others who behave like you. What is there to do? He should not make me jealous. He should not keep looking around. He should pay attention to me. He should not go anywhere without telling me.*

Impassive: *Your problem is not his going somewhere without telling you. You don't want him to go anywhere at all without you—if possible, not even to work, or you want him to work somewhere where only men are employed. What was it the other day? You were even jealous of his sister. The girl had a problem and she will of course talk with her brother. You are sometimes jealous of his cousins too. You really gave him hell for going on a trip with them during the last holiday. On the top of it, his cousins and you know each other very well.*

Jealous: *Well, fine, if they know me why I didn't go with them. What could I have done to them? If he didn't take me on that trip, he surely had something malicious in his mind.*

Impassive: *Of course, he won't take you; remember what you did the last time. You made remarks about their bathing suits, you made remarks about their dancing, and you did not leave them in peace. Didn't he say to you, "I will never go on holiday with you again"? Did you change your behavior at all? If I was going on a trip with him, I would just enjoy the holiday, and say "Oh! How nice to be on holiday with you." Instead of caring about the bathing suits of other girls or bothering about who he is dancing with, I would focus on how I would enjoy myself. You don't even know how to have fun. What do you want?*

Jealous: *I want to feel loved. I am afraid of being alone, all by myself.* (She starts to cry.) *You know that I don't really* *have anybody else. I don't want to be alone. I am so scared of being by myself. I keep thinking that he is going to leave me and I am horrified.* (Her crying increases.) *I can't be like you. If I am, he will leave.*

Impassive: *To tell the truth, I don't want to be alone either, but if he goes, he goes. If you ask me, he has no intention of leaving; otherwise he would have left already. But he is fed up with you, he can't breathe. Why do you think he doesn't worry about your leaving him?*

Jealous: *How can I? I can't live without him, all alone . . .*

Impassive: *You are obsessed with this "all alone" thing. What does that mean? Sometimes people can be by themselves. But yours is not a being-by-yourself issue. You are worried about being without a man. What if you did not have a boyfriend? I am really pissed off with you.* (While she was saying this, her voice was raised; she was breathing more rapidly, and her fists were clenched.)

As can be seen from the dialogue, Ruth eventually became more aware of the side that she named impassive, and she became able to express the feelings and thoughts of that side more easily. As the dialogue progressed, her existential impasse about "being all alone" became apparent. During the following part of the therapy, work was carried out on the introjected messages that were at the base of her existential anxieties.

In conclusion, working with resistance in therapy requires great sensitivity and a high level of skill. While on one hand, the therapist has to respect and appreciate the client's resistance; on the other hand, he/she also has to help him/her to overcome it. At the end of this work, the client will be able to accept his/her resistance, to discover its meaning and purpose, to confront it, and to integrate it within his/her personality. In this way, he/she will be ready to change.

17

BODY LANGUAGE

The most significant characteristic of the Gestalt approach that distinguishes it from other therapy approaches is the importance it gives to body language and the way it handles body-related clues.

Perls was very much influenced by his analyst Reich, who was both a psychoanalyst and a body therapist, and also by the points of view of the theater director Max Reinhardt and the dancer Palucca (Clarkson and Mackewn 1993, 40) on expressing feelings and thoughts through the body. This led him to give particular emphasis on body work in therapy. In the Gestalt approach, it is possible to group the body-related clues into three groups, which are as follows:

a. Facial expression, eye contact, changes in voice, and gestures

b. Movements of various parts of the body (e.g., tapping the foot, wringing the hands) and physical clues (e.g., pain, ache, breath holding)

c. Body structure and posture

Before mentioning how these body-related clues are handled in therapy, it will be worthwhile to look at the fundamental perspectives that underlie this emphasis on body language in the Gestalt approach.

Fundamental Perspectives of Body Work

Bodily, Emotional, and Mental Processes Function as a Whole

According to the Gestalt approach, the person is a whole with his/her body, thoughts, and feelings. In other words, body, mind, and soul are different aspects of the person, and thus they function as a whole (Mackewn 1999, 159). For example, when we are maltreated by someone, we get angry, and in responding to that person, our voice becomes higher, our body tenses and our fists clench; on the other hand, when we come across someone we like on the street, we start smiling and move forward to shake his/her hand or kiss him/her, and we speak in a soft tone. In such situations the body, mind, and soul are in harmony and reflect the existence style of the person at that moment. However, in some situations, disharmony between the body, mind, and soul can be observed. For example, although a person feels angry with someone who has maltreated him/her, he/she may not be aware of this anger because of his/her belief that getting angry is a negative thing and may even claim that he/she feels calm. But the feeling of anger can manifest itself as a headache even though he/she is neither aware of it nor accepting it. A person who is feeling alone may try not to be aware of this feeling as he/she does not know how to deal with this loneliness and may desensitize and stress him/herself by tensing the shoulder and chest muscles in particular. According to the Gestalt approach, dis-ease between the body, mind, and soul, or in other words between the body, thought, and feeling, can lead to a multitude of problems from desensitization to psychosis and can also cause deterioration of the physical health. In the emergence of the disharmony or dis-ease among the body, mind, and soul unfinished business, poles, resistances, and unhealthy use of contact styles can play important roles.

The Meaning of Bodily Reactions, Physical Symptoms, and Body Structure Is Unique for Each Person

According to the Gestalt approach, the meaning of a person's bodily movements at a particular moment is specific to that moment and to that person. For example, a person may tilt his/her head sideways when feeling sad, someone else when feeling helpless, and another when feeling angry; or a person may cross his/her arms sometimes to feel safe and secure and sometimes to show his/her self-confidence. Again, the meaning of the physical symptoms experienced by a person can differ from person to person or for the same person from time to time. We may hold our breath sometimes in order not to be aware of feelings, sometimes not to tell our inner thoughts and sometimes because of our excitement. Our headaches may sometimes be due to our dissatisfaction with ourselves, sometimes due to our dissatisfaction with others or with a particular situation. Similarly, some of us may take up a position as if hiding our head between our shoulders in order not to be seen by others, some of us not to see others. Some of us might make a habit of walking with a very straight back to avoid aggressive behavior toward others, some of us to protect ourselves from the aggressive behavior of others and some of us because of being very rigid emotionally. As can be understood from all these examples, what each person's body says (his/her body language) has a unique meaning and only the person him/herself can know what that meaning is. Thus, according to the Gestalt approach, the interpretation or assignation of certain meanings to one's body language by another person is totally wrong. In recent years, body language has started to be embraced by other therapy approaches, and books have started to appear on the subject. However, in some of the publications in this field, certain body movements or postures are presented as having the same meaning for everybody. According to some, for example, if a person crosses his/her arms while talking, it means that he/she is not open to communication, or tapping one's foot during a conversation indicates uneasiness. The Gestalt approach is totally against such interpretations or generalizations.

Spontaneous Body Reactions Reflect the Truth

In social life, people are mostly interested in what the person is saying; that is, they are concerned with the content of what is being said. Less attention is given to how it is said and the body movements accompanying the speech. In other words, in daily communication, the language a person uses "verbally" is given greater importance than the "body" language. Especially in our age, where intellect, logic, and knowledge are of particular value, the body receives attention only in terms of physical health and appearance. However, researchers have indicated that, even if not noticed consciously, as much as two-thirds of interpersonal communication is relayed nonverbally (Passons 1975, 101). While we talk, our body spontaneously accompanies our speech. In most cases, this is not planned or done with a purpose. Raising our eyebrows and opening our mouths when we are surprised, our rock-hard body when we are obliged to hug somebody we don't like, and our soft and melodic voices when we caress a baby are all spontaneous. They are very hard to control. On the other hand, we almost always preplan what we are going to say and try to control what is to be uttered. From time to time, we might choose to lie or to hide the truth. However, our bodily reactions inevitably "leak" to the outside, and whether this leakage is a vague gesture or a very obvious hand movement, it is still significant (Passons 1975, 102). Hence bodily reactions, which are an indicator of our feeling and thoughts at that particular moment, reflect the truth much more fully than what we are saying. In other words, they show "what we actually want to say." Simkin (1974, 3) calls the bodily and nonverbal reactions as "truth buttons."

Yontef (1993, 61) and Mackewn (1996, 164) have pointed out that feelings are generally experienced in and through the body, and hence, in the understanding of feelings in particular, bodily reactions are more reliable than verbal messages. There are also many expressions we use in our daily language that show that feelings are experienced in and through the body. For example, while expressions such as sending chills down one's spine, to make one's hair curl, and to make one's blood run cold are used to describe being scared of something or someone; breathtaking or spine-tingling are used for excitement.

How to Work with Body Language in Therapy

The purpose of body work carried out during therapy is to help the client to be able (a) to become aware of his/her own body, posture, bodily reactions, and physical ailments, (b) to discover what they mean for him/her, and (c) to ensure the integrity of body, mind, and emotions. There are many methods that can be used in therapy to reach these goals. To facilitate comprehensibility, possible body-related therapeutic interventions are presented under the groups of body reactions emerging during therapy, physical ailments, body structure, and posture. However, before going into therapeutic interventions, it will be useful to touch upon some points that are common in all body language related work in the Gestalt approach.

According to the Gestalt approach, not being aware of the sensations of certain parts or functions of one's body is to remain out of contact with important parts of oneself (Polster and Polster 1974, 115). As bodily reactions spontaneously accompany the person's thoughts and feelings, a person who is not aware of his/her body cannot be aware of his/her feelings and thoughts either. Gaining an awareness of bodily processes during therapy helps in getting to the roots of the main problems of that person more quickly. In order to heighten bodily awareness, the therapist has to be a very good observer. Perls et al. (1951/1996), in order to underline the importance of this, stated that the Gestalt approach actually focuses on the obvious. The therapist should continuously be aware of the client's body and bodily reactions during the therapy and, when it is considered helpful, should transmit his/her observations to the client (Mackewn 1997, 45). However, before sharing his/her observations regarding the body and the bodily reactions of the client, the therapist should give information to the client about issues such as body-mind-soul integration, the importance of the body and bodily expressions, the benefits of being aware of them and discovering their meaning. Otherwise, the therapist will not only be obstructing the physical, intellectual, and emotional processes of the client but might cause him/her to feel embarrassed.

As already mentioned, Reich's body armour concept greatly influenced the body work in the Gestalt approach. The part of Reich's perspective that influenced Perls most was his view that "the characteristics which can be physically observed in a person's body are indicators of his/her inner existence." However, the way body language work is carried out in the Gestalt approach differs significantly from Reich's method. According to Reich (1945/1972, 270) people try to block their unacceptable emotional reactions by tensing or compressing certain muscle groups in their body. If this becomes chronic, then the tenseness in the muscles become permanent and covers the person's body like armour and affects his/her posture. The eyes, mouth, neck, chest, stomach, and hips are the parts of the body that are most affected by this. According to this perspective, the energy that was entrapped in the body and constituted the body armour, or in other words the resistance, has to be released as soon as possible. In the Reich approach, in therapy, first, the muscle groups causing the formation of this body armour are determined, and then the tension and compression in the muscles are relieved through relaxation exercises and pressure applications, and later the psychological conflicts are analyzed. In contrast to this, in the Gestalt approach, instead of instantly getting rid of bodily symptoms, reactions, or posture, it is believed that it is necessary first to own and to be aware of them fully, as otherwise it will not be possible to define the meaning of these bodily reactions.

How to Work with Body Reactions that Emerge in Therapy

The work done regarding the bodily reactions emerging in the session can be grouped under two headings: raising the awareness of bodily reactions and exploring the meaning of the reactions.

Raising the Awareness of Bodily Reactions

One of the most important tasks of the therapist related to body language is to help the client to be aware of his/her bodily reactions emerging in the session. For this, first the therapist has to be aware of all the bodily reactions of the client. However, the therapist does not share all of his/her observations with the client. Passing on every observation to the client can lead to a feeling of being under constant observation and unease in the client and can also make him/her unable to tell all he/ she wants to tell. Hence, the therapist has to be selective about which observations will be shared. While making such a selection, the following criteria should be applied.

- *When what the client says and his/her nonverbal reactions are not compatible.* When what the client says and his/her nonverbal behavior are compatible, for example, if the client says that he/she is angry and at the same time he/she is knitting his/her brows and his/her voice is high, then there is no need to give feedback since the person is reacting as a whole with his/her feelings, thoughts, and body. On the other hand, if the client is jiggling his/her leg while talking about a pleasant memory with his/her mother, if the client uses a very monotonous voice while talking about being angry or tenses his/her neck and shoulders while saying that he/she is feeling at ease; that is, if the spoken statements and nonverbal reactions are not compatible, then the therapist can mention these observations to the client. In such cases there is a conflict, a split between the body, feelings, and thought of the client and the person is not reacting as a whole.

- *When the client remains silent.* When a client sits without uttering a word, it does not mean that he/she is not thinking about anything or is feeling nothing, but it indicates that he/she is experiencing something but not expressing it. There may be many reasons for the client's not expressing his/her thoughts and feelings. For example, the client might be bored, scared, angry, disappointed, upset, anxious, or ashamed. In cases where the client remains silent, if the therapist observes a certain reaction in his/her body, then the therapist can inform the client about these observations. For example, the therapist can help the client to be aware of his/her feelings and thoughts with remarks such as "I notice that you have been staring at the floor for some time," "I see that you are playing with your hands," or "I realize that you are overtensing your legs."

- *When a change occurs in the behavior or attitude of the client.* The therapist must also be aware of the emerging changes in the behavior and attitude of the client. For example, when a client who always sits on the same chair sits in a different one, when one who always dresses in dark colors starts to dress colorfully, when there is a change in his/her hair or beard or mustache, when the ones who always avoid eye contact start making contact, or when a chronic low-voiced speaker starts to speak more loudly, the therapist can share his/her observations and explore what these changes mean for the client.

While sharing his/her observations that are based on the aforementioned criteria, in order to be able to help the client to be aware of his/her body or in other words to be aware of him/herself, the therapist should pay attention to the following parts and features of the body:

Head. Head movements are significant in communication. In daily communications, for example, the right-left movement of the head means "no," while the up-down movement means "yes." Other than these general meanings, the head movements of the client during therapy have meanings that are specific to that person. Hence, the therapist can convey his/her observations by saying, "I see that you are holding your head very tensely" or "I am aware that you keep your head lowered" and can go into investigating the meaning of such behavior.

Mouth and jaw. The mouth and jaw are important in terms of expressing feelings. This area can give clues about feelings such as sadness, happiness, joy, or about self-harming behaviors (biting the lips) or self-protection (keeping the lips tightly closed). The reason why clowns, actors, dancers, and mime artists paint or cover their mouth and jaw area is because they do not want to show their true feelings. The therapist can try to raise the client's awareness with remarks such as "I saw you smiling slightly," "I am aware that you are moving your lips," or "I see that you are tensing your jaws."

Voice and manner of speaking. How something is said is as important as what is being said. Hence, while the therapist is listening to the client, he/she needs to develop a "third" ear. In this way, the therapist can lead the client's attention to his/her voice or manner of speech with remarks such as "Your voice is becoming gradually lower," "Your voice has risen and become high-pitched," "I realize that you are speaking more rapidly," or "I see that you are passing on to another sentence without finishing your first."

Eyes and eyebrows. Eyes and eyebrows are the areas where feelings such as self-protection, anger, sadness, joy, love, surprise, or fear are mostly reflected. Furthermore, whether or not the client is keeping eye contact with the therapist may give significant clues about the client-therapist relation. The therapist can give feedback to the client with remarks such as "I see that you are blinking rapidly," "I see your pupils have enlarged," "I am aware that you have not been looking at me for a while," "I recognize that you are knitting your brows," or "I see that you are raising your eyebrows frequently."

Nose. Initially one might think that the nose does not have a significant role in expressing feelings, but a closer look shows that there are many sayings and expressions in our daily life that involve the nose such as "having one's nose up in the air" or "sticking one's nose into everything," "keeping one's nose out of something," or "it's no skin off my nose." Comments such as "I am aware that your nose is getting red," "I see your nostrils are expanding," "I realize that you are breathing through your nose" may be used to increase the client's awareness.

Neck and shoulders. The area where tension is most frequently and most strongly experienced is the neck and shoulders. This area is also important for the movement of the arms. Expressions such as "I see that you are hunching your shoulders," "I am aware that you are pushing your shoulders back," or "I see that you are keeping your neck very straight" can help the client to gain awareness.

Arms and hands. Arms and hands generally accompany speech. Some people even believe that without their arms and hands they can never fully express themselves. However, some others find hand and arm movements made while speaking very annoying as they distract them from focusing on what is being said. The therapist can attract the client's attention to his/her arms and hands with remarks and questions such as "I see that you have clenched your fists," "I am aware that your arms are crossed on your chest," or "Are you aware of what your fingers are doing at this moment?"

Legs and feet. Legs and feet have three basic functions. The first of these is to carry the upper part of the body, the second is self-protection, and the third is to enable the whole body to move. Hence, the legs can be informative in many ways. The client could be made aware of his/her legs and feet with remarks and questions such as "I am aware that you are jiggling your right leg," "Are you aware of what are your feet doing just now?" or "I see that you are continuously changing the position of your legs."

Whole body. The posture of the body itself can also provide clues about feelings. Observations such as "I see that you are sitting on the edge of the couch," "I am aware that you are rocking your body," or "You leaned all the way forward while saying this" can help the client to focus on his/her body. Furthermore, the sensations such as acceleration of the heartbeat, heartburn, or increased bowel movement, which cannot be seen externally but experienced internally, can also be related with feelings. In order to help the client to be aware of these sensations, the therapist from time to time could ask, "What is happening in your body just now?"

Autonomic reactions. During therapy autonomic reactions such as sweating, blushing, itching, twitching, feeling cold, shaking, flushing should also be noticed. The therapist can heighten the client's awareness with comments such as "I see that your face is blushing," "I am aware that your eye is twitching," or "You seem to be shivering."

Manner of breathing. In the Gestalt approach, the manner of breathing is considered to be very important as it is believed that the way a person breathes affects that person's feelings, interpretations, and his/her worldview, that is, his/her experiences from moment to moment. When we change the way we breathe, when we hold our breath, breathe rapidly, or take shallow or deep breaths, we also change our emotional or physiological state. For example, when we hold our breath, we don't just lose our voice, we also lose our feelings. That is, we don't feel anything, and we are not aware of the here and now. Awareness of manner of breathing is especially significant in terms of anxiety disorders. Furthermore, it is possible to summarize the therapy of this disorder with the slogan "inhale-exhale and act" (Daş 2004). The therapist can support the client in increasing his/her awareness regarding the way he/she breathes with remarks such as "I see that you are holding your breath," "I notice that you are breathing rapidly," "I am aware that you have taken a deep breath."

Exploring the Meaning of Bodily Reactions

in Therapy

During therapy, various ways can be utilized to explore the meaning of the bodily and nonverbal reactions of the client. Some of these are given below.

Exaggeration

While employing this technique, the client is asked to exaggerate as much as possible the bodily movement he/she is doing at that moment. Exaggeration is a very effective method in becoming aware of certain feelings that otherwise could be missed or in recalling some memories. For example, Sue was talking in a very low voice while she was discussing her relationship with her husband. When she was asked to talk in an even lower voice, she realized how much she actually was afraid of her husband. John, while talking about how beneficial it would be for him to go abroad for his training, was swinging his leg back and forth. When he was asked to exaggerate this movement, John started swinging his leg higher and faster and realized that his leg looked "as if it were kicking something." While searching for what he might want to kick, he suddenly said "the ball" and remembered that he had attended a football school during the summer when he was about nine or ten years old. That summer, although he wanted to go on a holiday with his mother, because of his father's insistence, he had to stay at home. His father insisted that he should attend the football school in the town. Furthermore, as he did not like it and was not good at playing football, he was frequently scolded by the coach and was very ashamed. His father was greatly disappointed by this and started to keep his distance from John. All this made John feel both very angry and sad, but he could not show his feelings to anybody. He was also feeling guilty for disappointing his father. At that time, he promised himself never to disappoint his father again and started to do whatever his father wanted exactly in the way he wanted. Going abroad for his training was also his father's idea. Even though John appeared as if he had convinced himself of the benefits of going abroad for his training, with the exaggeration of his leg swinging, he realized how angry he was with his father and that he actually did not want to go.

Doing the Opposite

In some cases, it might be useful to want the client to do exactly the opposite of whatever he/she is doing at that moment to foster awareness of his/her feelings and needs. For example, Anne was talking in a very monotonous tone of voice about an incident at work, and she was sitting hunched over. When asked how she was feeling about this incident, her reply was "I don't know." Then she was asked to tell the same incident with opened-up shoulders and in a more lively tone of voice. During this second narration, Anne realized how much her boss looked like her father and how much afraid she was of him because of this. While carrying out "doing the opposite" experiments, the client can be asked to repeat the opposing movements over and over again and, while doing so, to focus on his/her feelings. For example, Terry, who kept talking with his head down, was asked to lift and then lower his head again and to repeat this several times. While performing this repetition several times, Terry realized that when his head was down he felt vulnerable and inadequate and more confident when his head was up.

Creating a Dialogue

In this experiment, the client can create a dialogue with various parts of his/her body (e.g., hand, leg, or heart) or a dialogue can be carried out among different parts of the body (e.g., one hand with the other, the upper part of the body with the lower).

For example, Andrew was struggling with a loss of sexual desire in his relationship with his wife. When talking about his unwillingness in the sexual relationship, Andrew was constantly holding his ear. Hence, Andrew was asked to create a dialogue between his hand and his ear.

Hand: *I am covering you and so I prevent you from hearing well.*

Therapist: *What in particular are you preventing him from hearing?*

Hand: *I don't know what exactly. Maybe hearing about sexual subjects.*

Therapist: *Say this to your ear.*

Hand: *I don't want you to hear anything about sex. That's why I am covering you.*

Ear:	*But I want to hear. Why don't you want me to hear?*
Hand:	*Because I am very much ashamed of this situation and of the fact that I have to talk about it.*
Ear:	*Are you ashamed of me?*
Hand:	*Both of you and of the ears of others. I don't want them to hear it.*
Therapist:	*Who especially do you not want to hear this?*
Hand:	*I don't know . . . everybody.*
Therapist:	*If you had to choose one person in particular, who would it be that makes you feel ashamed?*
Hand:	*My father.*

During the rest of the session, his father's scornful remarks about his "masculinity" were revealed and the effects of these remarks on Andrew were explored.

How to Work with Physical Disturbances in Therapy

In the Gestalt approach, one of the areas of interest is bodily disturbances. Examples of bodily disturbances may be problems such as pain, hurt, cramping, burning, or swelling, as well as all psychosomatic disturbances.

The Gestalt approach believes that all these problems have a functional meaning for the person concerned and they actually give messages to that person about his/her needs, even though they have not yet been recognized by the person. Hence, during the therapy, some work is carried out to reveal the meaning of bodily disturbances for the client and the messages they are trying to convey (Clarkson 1991, 22). Below, some of the techniques that could be utilized during such work are presented.

Owning the Body

This experiment starts with asking the client to change his/her statements about body-related disturbances into the "I" form in order to enable him/her to own them. For example, when the client says, "My head is aching," he/she is asked to change it to, "I am aching"; the client who says, "My ears do not hear," is asked to change it to "I am not hearing," or "I am shallow" replaces "My breath is shallow." By altering these expressions, the client can understand that such symptoms do not appear spontaneously or independently of him/herself and start taking responsibility for them. After the changing of the expressions into the "I" form, than it is possible to move into the exploration of the meaning of the relevant disturbance. An example of how such an experiment can be carried out is given below.

Kerry : *Right now it feels as if my jaw is locked.*

Therapist : *Can you change this into "I am locking up" and say it.*

Kerry : *I am locking up.*

Therapist : *Who is locking you up?*

Kerry : *Nobody, how would I know* (His voice is lowered and he tears up). (After a long silence) *When I was little, my mother used to lock me up in the bathroom, but I didn't think about it for a long time.*

Therapist : *What used to happen?*

Kerry : *When I misbehaved, when I made my mother angry, she used to shut me in the bathroom. It would be very dark, and I would be very scared. I used to scream, "Let me out," but she would say that for each scream, she would keep me in there ten minutes longer. Then I would be quiet and cry. She would be very angry when I cried too. Sometimes she would deride me, calling me "sissy." This would make me feel awful.* (Tearing up again, his lip starts to quiver, and he stops talking.)

Therapist : *What are you locking up right now? I see you are getting teary and you are not talking.*

Kerry : *I don't know. Maybe I am locking up my voice and my tears.*

Therapist : *I am aware that you are holding your breath. Take a breath.*

Kerry : (Starts to cry and it went goes on for some time)

Therapist : *It looks as if you have unlocked your tears. Now unlock your voice. Scream, "Let me out."*

Kerry : *Let me out.*

Therapist : *Louder.*

Kerry : (A little louder) *Let me out.*

Therapist : *Louder.*

Kerry : (Really loud and crying) *Leet meee ouuut!*

Later, to facilitate the completion of this unfinished business of Kerry and his mother, two-chair work was carried out.

Intensifying the Disturbance

In this experiment, the client is asked to increase the physical disturbance he/she experiences in his/her body, to feel it fully, and to articulate it. Such a practice can help the client to become aware of his/her feelings, such as anger, sadness, guilt, anxiety, and the like, related to the disturbance he/she is experiencing, and this helps in recalling memories that are connected with these feelings. Below is a part of a very long and emotionally intensive session with a client who was complaining about chronic back pain and headaches.

Joe : *My back is very painful today.*

Therapist : *Feel the pain fully and try to intensify it. How can you do that?*

Joe : *When I tense my back muscles more, the pain increases.*

Therapist : OK. *Tense your back muscles more, increase the pain, and make a sound to express the pain.*

Joe : *Agh!*

Therapist : *Louder and longer.*

Joe : *Aggghh.*

Therapist : *Carry on. One right after the other, don't stop. Louder and longer.*

Joe :	*Aaaaggghhhh. Aaaaagggggghhh. Aaaaaaagggggghhhhhh!* (He starts to get more and more angry, and his voice becomes louder.)
Therapist :	*What are you feeling right now?*
Joe :	*I am very angry, damn it.*
Therapist :	*Who are you angry with?*
Joe :	*I don't know. I am just angry.*
Therapist :	*Keep increasing the pain by tensing your muscles and shouting to express the pain.*
Joe :	*It is very painful. Aaaaaaaagggggghhhhhh.*
Therapist :	*I see that you are pushing your shoulders and arms back when you are tensing your back muscles. Do these more, push them further back, and make sounds to express the pain.*
Joe :	(pushing back) *Aaaaaagggghhhhhh.*
Therapist :	*What happens to your arms when you do this?*
Joe :	*I am immobilizing them.*
Therapist :	*Make them even more immobilized. What can you not do with your arms in this position?*
Joe :	*I can't hit, I can't push, and I can't throw anything* (just then his voice lowers and he starts to stare at the floor).
Therapist :	*What is happening just now?*
Joe :	*I just had a vision* (with a very sad tone of voice and facial expression). *My father, mother, and me. We are eating. My mother and father are talking, and I am watching the television. I have the TV remote in my hand. I don't know why, but suddenly, I realize that my mother and father are arguing. My father is shouting at my mother, and my mother is both crying and shouting back. My father becomes more and more angry, grabs the remote I had put on the table, and throws it at my mother. It hits my mother in the face, and her face is all bloody.*
Therapist :	*What are you feeling now?*
Joe :	(sobbing) *I am very sorry, and I feel guilty.*
Therapist :	*Guilty of what?*

Joe :	*Putting the remote on the table. If I hadn't left it there, then my father could not have thrown it at my mother.*
Therapist :	*What are your feelings for your father?*
Joe :	*I am very angry with him, but there is nothing I can do.* He beats me too. My back is aching terribly.
Therapist :	*Intensify the pain and keep making the sounds.*

As the session progressed, Joe started to see the connections between his back pain and his unexpressed anger toward his father. There is no doubt that what was revealed during this session was not the single cause of Joe's back pains. In later sessions, work was carried out on other memories and feelings that could be related to these pains.

Acceptance of the Disturbance

This work helps the client to accept the situation and to reorganize his/her life in cases of incurable illnesses (e.g., diabetes, rheumatoid arthritis), organ loss (e.g., kidney removal, severed arm), or loss of function (e.g., being sterile, paralysis of a leg) instead of living with sustained negative feelings and a sense of incompleteness. However, before starting such an experiment, the client should have experienced all the angers, anxieties, fears, and sorrows related to his/her situation during the therapy; his/her conflicts should be solved, and all unfinished business should be completed. Such an experiment should never be carried out until the client is ready, and he/she should never be rushed. Work related to the acceptance of the disturbance is generally carried out with the empty-chair technique. In empty-chair practice, the problem—be it diabetes, the single kidney, the severed arm, the ovaries, which caused infertility—"sit" on the empty chair, and the client is requested to talk to the disturbance on the chair and explain that he/she is ready to live with it. Even though this type of work generally leads to the experiencing of deep sorrows, they are nevertheless very helpful in enabling the client to achieve a creative adjustment. Judith, who was a multiple sclerosis patient, during the experiment concerning the acceptance of the disturbance, talked in tears to her illness in the following way:

Judith: *It was very hard for me to accept you. You know that for months I did not want to accept you. I hated you. I was ashamed of you, I was afraid of you, I was very anxious because of you. Because of you, I did not want to talk to anybody. I even thought that you were sent to me as some sort of punishment. I kept asking "why me?" I still don't have the answer to this question. Sometimes you hinder me so much. You hurt me, leave me in pain, and make me writhe in agony. Sometimes, I fell so helpless that I cry for hours. I don't even want to live any longer because of you. I rebel against everything, against everybody. So many times I cursed the doctors for not helping me. So many times I swore and cursed them. Then I pitied myself a lot. How I put myself down. I felt incomplete, inadequate, ugly, but most important of all, I felt vile. But I finally understood that I cannot get rid of you. You are part of me and I accept you. Of course I am not very happy to be with you, but I also know that the more I hate you the more distress you cause me. The other day, I even managed to laugh in spite of you. I especially like my friends at the new course I am attending. I haven't mentioned you to them yet, but when the time comes I will. I will not be ashamed of you and I will not pity myself. I hope you don't progress too rapidly; you will not invade all my muscles and be fair. I hope you don't disfigure me too much either. Maybe they can discover new remedies soon, but no matter what happens, we will obviously end this life together. Yes, I accept you, and I want to live long and happily with you for as long as possible. Oh yes, there is something else, even though I never wanted to learn it this way and from you, but thanks to you I learned to be patient, to be resilient, strong, and determined. I want to teach what I have learned to others, but please leave it to me and don't make them sick, don't try to teach them the way you thought me. Let me be the one to teach them, please!*

How to Work with Body Structure and Posture in Therapy

Some of us keep our shoulders down and forward and keep our body hunched. Some of us walk very upright; some of us walk holding our upper body back while others hold back the lower part. In some of us, the upper body looks as if loaded on top of the lower part. Some of us stand with our chest pushed forward while others lead with their bellies. Some of us swing from side to side while walking or walk with our feet apart. All these postures and those not mentioned here are determined by our genetic characteristics and habits we have made while striving to adjust to life. In other words, our body structure and posture is the end result of the creative adjustment we have made to survive in our environment, in addition to our genetic characteristics (Kepner 1987, 49).

During the evolution of the creative adjustment, we tend to adopt certain postures more frequently, according to the feelings we experience in our environment. For example, a child who frequently witnesses arguments in the family within which he/she is growing up, fearing the arguments and their consequences, might want not to hear them and try to hide his/her ears by moving his/her head down to the shoulders. Or a child who is constantly harassed by other children, in order to protect him/herself and scare the others, might develop a straight and tense posture with one shoulder kept high and forward, a posture popularly known as "rowdy." Another child who is frequently criticized, no matter how angry and sad he/she feels because of these criticisms, realizing that revealing these feelings to those who criticize him/her will lead to much worse consequences, may make a habit of holding his/her breath and pulling his/her belly in for not feeling anything. It is possible to multiply these examples further. However, what is being emphasized here is the fact that when faced with the same situation frequently, the child becomes used to holding a certain position, and as time passes, the muscles start to retain the position permanently. Consequently, even though there are no longer arguing parents, harassing children, or critical people around him/her, the child keeps sustaining that position. In the end, it becomes his/her posture in life and becomes fixed.

When body position and posture are fixed, then adopting any other position becomes very difficult for that person (Kepner 1987, 51). For example, a person who has made a habit of hunching up and hiding his/her head between his/her shoulders will have great difficulty in holding the head up and shoulders down. It will be also very difficult and disturbing for one with a "rowdy" posture trying to hold the shoulders aligned and relax his/her body or for one who usually holds his/her breath and pulls the belly in, not to do this. In time, a person might not even be aware of the abnormality of his/her posture.

The aim of work related to body structure and posture during therapy is to reach an awareness of this fixed body structure, to discover its meaning, and to achieve integration of the body, feelings, thoughts, and behavior (Kepner 1987, 52). For this purpose, the following exercises can be used in therapy.

Becoming Aware of the Position

One of the ways of making a client aware of the position would be to ask the client to look at his/her posture in the mirror. Another way to help the client to be aware of different parts of his/her body can be to ask the client to lie on the floor and check the different parts of his/her body that are not resting naturally (e.g., bent into a certain direction, turned inward or outward, not fully touching the floor). Later by exaggerating the postures that the client became aware of while looking in the mirror or lying down, the client's full awareness of his/her body structure and posture is achieved. These types of experiments are the first steps of accepting and owning the body structure and posture as the client now takes this position consciously whereas he/she had been holding this posture unaware for years.

Discovering the Meaning of the Position

For this, the client can be asked to show both the position recognized while looking in the mirror or while lying on the floor and its exact opposite in an exaggerated way. For example, he/she can be asked to repeat several times the position of hiding the head between the shoulders and the position of pushing the head upward, which enables the head to move easily. Meanwhile, the feelings and thoughts of the client while holding the different positions can be worked on. Here, the therapist helps the client to find a sentence for each position that describes the meaning the positions have for him/her. One example is that for Linda, who was hunched and hiding her head between her shoulders, the meaning of this posture was "Don't see me, don't look at me" and "I don't want to look at you and to see you either." For Linda, the position where she was not hiding her head but moving it freely meant "Look at me, see me" and "I also want to see you and to look at you."

Developing a New Theme from the Position

The purpose of work carried out at this stage is, after discovering the meaning or in other words the theme of body structure and posture, to change this theme and integrate it into the personality. During these experiments, the goal is not to change the body structure or posture but to carry out deeper and integrating work on the defined theme. For this, various methods can be used in therapy. One of them is the phenomenological research method. For example, when Linda was asked, "What happens if they look at you or see you?" her reply was along the lines of "They won't like me," "They won't think I am nice," "They will think that I made a mistake." Her reply when asked, "What happens if you see them or look at them?" was "I would see that they did not like me, did not think I was nice, and then I would be very sorry and may be very angry." Obviously all these replies were related to such introjected messages as "making mistakes, not to be liked, not to be considered nice." Once these themes were determined, then work was carried out on Linda's introjected messages. One of the ways that can be used during work on developing a new theme could be creating a dialogue among these two parties of "see me" and "don't see me" by using a two-chair technique.

In conclusion, Gestalt therapy—by focusing on the body, bodily reactions, bodily disturbances, and posture and offering various methods for working on them—greatly contributes to the field of psychology. The fact that the client him/herself finds out the meaning of his/her body language during therapy enables the client to establish the connection between his/her body, feelings, thoughts, and behavior and to integrate them more easily. However, as body-related work is completely unfamiliar to the client, it can lead to the experiencing of deep shame, so it should only be carried out after a satisfactory therapist- client relation is established and by a creative and experienced therapist who is aware of his/her own body language.

18

DREAMS

In general, one-third of our life is spent in sleep. Sleep is not a passive slowing down in the functions of the organism or a passing into stillness, but it is, on the contrary, an active process. Studies in the field of sleep physiology have revealed that sleep has two physiological states: REM and non-REM (Özer 2003). During sleep these two physiological states cyclically follow each other. Dreams emerge in the REM phase. Immediately after falling asleep, the non-REM phase starts, and approximately 90–100 minutes later, the sleeper goes into the REM phase where dreaming starts. While the REM phase is about 5–10 minutes during the first hours of sleep, it can go up to 20–40 minutes in the later hours. Hence, most of the dreams are in the last one-third of sleep. REM sleep is approximately 15–20 percent of the total sleep time (Shapiro and Flanigan 1993, 5). Generally even though there are four or five dreams in seven or eight hours of sleep, many people remember those that are close to waking up, that is, toward morning.

While reading these lines, you might think, "I have had no dreams recently" or "I seldom dream." However, when looked in the light of the above information, it is not true to say, "I don't dream," the truth is that you do not remember them. The contents of the dreams can vary. Some dreams are related to daily situations. While some draw your attention to something you have forgotten, others may be intended to solve a persistent problem. Some dreams emphasize feelings such as anger, worry, or fear, while others can bring forth sexuality. There can be also future-related dreams or dreams that prepare the person for the future. Again, some dreams could be about the meaning of your life or some social or cultural characteristics. We can easily multiply these examples. According to Latner (1992), whatever their content is, spontaneously occurring dreams can help us to understand ourselves much better than we can when we are awake. (Perls 1969, 145) has also stated that dreams are the most spontaneous expressions of a person's existence, and problems related to the existence of any individual are most clearly came in view in his/her dreams.

Since 1960's there are many studies that show the importance of the dreams in terms of psychological and physiological health. For example, in a study carried out by Dement (1960) during the whole night, people were awakened just as they were about to dream and then they were allowed to go back to sleep. Despite the fact these people slept as many hours as they did on a regular basis, the next day, it was observed that they were functioning at a lower level, were in a low mood, and were eating more than they normally did. When this practice was carried out for several nights, a significant level of restlessness and anxiety was observed in those people.

Meaning of Dreams

The meanings of dreams are always covert; that is, it is impossible to discover their meanings without working on them. In other words, the dreams whose meanings are not understood are like unopened letters. According to the Gestalt approach that has an existentialist and phenomenological basis, the meaning of a dream is special to the dreamer and to his/her phenomenological field; hence it is specific to that person. Only the dreamer can know the meaning of something seen in a dream, and only that person can work it out (Downing and Marmorstein 1997, XVI). Nobody, other than the dreamer, can interpret a dream since the meaning of an element of the dream can vary from person to person. For example, everybody can dream about washing his/her face and drying it with a red towel. Such a dream may carry an existential message related to "cleaning" for the dreamer, while it may for somebody else reflect unclear aspects of the dreamer's personality, and for yet another, it may be an indicator of anger against the mother. Furthermore, when the same person has this same dream some other night, its meaning could be different from the previous one because everything in a dream is affected by that person's impressions, memories, thoughts, feelings, attitudes, attributions, and needs related to what he/she sees at that particular time.

When seen from this perspective, the viewpoints of the Gestalt approach related with the meanings of dreams significantly differ from those of other therapeutic approaches in general and from the psychoanalytical approach in particular. In the psychoanalytic approach, it is believed that whatever is seen in a dream carries the same meaning for everybody, and the therapist interprets the person's dream according to the meanings defined by the theory. Aside from the psychoanalytic approach, there are many views that elaborate upon the meaning of what is seen in dreams. There are even many books published under the title, "Dream Interpretations." For example, you might discover in such books that water in a dream is sexually related and the color red indicates generosity (Downing and Marmorstein 1997, XIII), whereas, in the Gestalt approach, it is believed that the meaning of a dream can never be discovered by the interpretations of the therapist and the explanations which are not specific to that person. Just like a poem, a painting, or a piece of music, a dream shows the worldview, feelings, and thoughts of the person creating it at the time it is created. In other words dreams give information about the person's form of existence.

The Aims of Dreamwork

According to the Gestalt approach, the aims of dreamwork are

a. To be aware of the rejected, disowned parts of the personality and to integrate those parts,

b. To be aware of the dreamer's needs and to find the meanings of existential messages,

c. To be aware of the dysfunctional contact styles in interpersonal relations and to change them.

Now, let us discuss them one by one.

a. To Be Aware of the Rejected, Disowned Parts of the Personality and to Integrate those Parts

According to Gestalt therapy, the most fundamental mechanism in dreams is projection (Frantz 1998, 47). In other words, the dream is a screen where the dreamer exhibits his or her projections. According to Perls (1969, 142), every element of a dream actually projects a characteristic related to our personality. Dreams cover both the accepted and the rejected, or in other words, owned or disowned parts of the personality. According to the Gestalt approach, the dreamer projects these rejected, disowned characteristics of his/her personality onto other people or objects in the dream, and thus believing that these characteristics belong to others, he/she feels relieved. Hence, it is difficult to accept that every object, person, situation, etc., we see in a dream actually projects a part of us; that is to say, they belong to us. However, no matter how difficult it is to accept, everything in a dream belongs to the dreamer because he/she is the one who is creating the dream. To give an example, let us assume that you dreamed you were swimming with your mother in a choppy sea on a sunny day. In this case, all the elements of the dream—the sun, the choppy sea, your mother, other swimmers, the island farther out and even the unseen but felt anxiety—reflect your characteristics. To give another example, let us say that you cannot fully remember your dream but only that there was a red car. This red car you dreamed about could be a wide, old, slow- moving car with partially peeling paint, or it could be, on the contrary, a new, modish, very quick, and very brightly painted car. It could be a car you used once or one you have never even been in. However, in the final say, all the features of this car show your positive or negative characteristics and tell you about yourself. In this sense, your dreams do not merely "belong" to you, but they are you, or you are your dreams. The rejected and disowned parts of the personality are no doubt most definitely experienced in nightmares (Perls 1969, 190). In nightmares anxiety and fear are the dominant feelings and there are voids, limitations, and inefficacies in the content of the dream that are difficult to comprehend. In nightmares, the rejected, disowned characteristics show themselves as bullies, monsters, wild animals, powerful creatures, extraterritorial events, accidents, illnesses, death, and the like, and in most cases, the dreamer faced with them feels weak and helpless and sees him/herself as an injured victim. According to the Gestalt approach, the armed men chasing you, the car with no brakes, the dog trying to bite you in the nightmare are all you; the one chased by the armed men, the one running from the car with no brakes, and the one who is bitten by the dog are also you. Hence, the nightmares signal the fact that it is time to bring some characteristics to light (Latner 1995/1996).

In the Gestalt approach, reaching an awareness of those parts that the person is rejecting, disowning, or in other words, of those parts he/she is projecting, is not enough: they also have to be integrated into the personality (Perls 1969, 120). Freud (1915) indicated that dreams are "a royal road to the subconscious," and he aimed in his dreamwork to bring the subconscious messages to the conscious. On the other hand, Perls (1969, 87) went a step further in his dreamwork and claimed that dreams are "a royal road to integration," and as long as integration is not achieved, the messages from the dreams will not contribute to growth and development. Moving on from this point of view, in Gestalt therapy dreamwork, the phases of experiencing, internalizing, and integrating the rejected and accepted sides and determining new goals are passed through. As the Gestalt approach believes that growth and development can only be achieved through integration, dreams that give messages about those parts of the personality that are not owned and thus not integrated are given much importance.

b. To Be Aware of the Needs and to Find the Meanings of Existential Messages

People have many needs that have to be met. As mentioned before, according to the Gestalt approach, the basis of the life is meeting the needs in the shortest time and by the easiest route (Serok 2000, 7–8). If a need is to be met, first it has to become clear, that is, it has to move from the background to become a distinct figure. When a need that has became a figure is satisfied, then it returns to the background, and a new need appears. However, if a need is not recognized, is not met because it is not accepted, or is blocked or repressed, then such a need can neither be turned into a distinct figure, nor can it move to the background completely. This prevents a new need from becoming a figure. In such cases, dreams can turn the person's attention to those needs that are significant in terms of his/her existence but which are ignored for various reasons (Fantz 1998, 46). When a need remains unsatisfied for a long time, then recurring dreams appear. Recurring dreams give messages that can help the person in becoming aware of what is missing in his/her life, the things the person is avoiding doing or experiencing, and what the person needs (Clarkson and Mackewn 1993, 120). For example, over the last year, Jill frequently dreamed about not being able to find her shoes or going out with an unmatched pair. In dreamwork, Jill realized that these recurring dreams were giving her a message about "putting on her shoes" and getting away from the unhappy relationship with her boyfriend that had been going on for two years. The dream also suggested that she needed another relationship that "matched"—that is, with someone better suited for her.

During dreamwork, after determining the needs that have been repressed or blocked, work is carried out on the feelings, thoughts, and beliefs related to that needs. For instance, as mentioned above, Jill was unaware of her need to break off her relationship, even though she was unhappy, because she was afraid of being alone, because she believed that she was getting too old for another relation, and because she thought that as she and her partner had been together for such a long time she had to stay with him. During therapy, after the determination of needs and the underlying thoughts, feelings, and beliefs, it is necessary to work on finding alternatives to meet those needs and developing environmental and personal support systems of the client.

c. To Be Aware of the Dysfunctional Contact Styles in Interpersonal Relations and to Change Them.

Another characteristic of dreams is that they inform the person about his/her unnoticed feelings and styles of contact regarding interpersonal relations. For example, a dream where you see your father coming toward you and then a pain starts in your chest can inform you about your feelings about your father of which you are unaware or about your contact style with him. In some cases, a dream may carry messages about thoughts that the client cannot freely talk about or feelings he/she could not properly express in therapy (Mackewn 1996, 148). Isadore From claims that dreams are "retroflected" messages sent to the therapist (referred to in Latner 1995/1996). Seeing the therapist in his/her dream is just as significant as not seeing the therapist at all in terms of giving clues regarding the client-therapist relationship and their contact style. For example, Adam dreamed about his therapist moving into the upper floor of his house. But later the therapist moved out because of the heating system that was not functioning properly. During the work on his dream, Adam realized that he actually wanted a "confluent" relationship with his therapist and was afraid that the therapist wouldn't find him "warm" and "loving" enough. During dreamwork, once awareness is achieved regarding the styles of contact used in interpersonal relations and the participants' feelings, then work is carried out to develop functional styles of contact.

Despite the fact that the aims of dreamwork in therapy were given under three subheadings, it is worthwhile not to view them as separate aims but rather as aims that complement each other. In other words, during dreamwork, while a single aim can be achieved, it is also possible to reach two or even three of the mentioned aims while working on the same dream. This means that, in some cases, by working on a single dream, it is possible to help the client to become aware of his/her rejected personality traits as well as his/her needs, feelings, and styles of contact.

Up to now, the aims of dreamwork and what can be done to reach them have been examined. Now, it is time to elaborate on "how" these goals can be achieved.

How to Work with Dreams in Therapy

Forgotten Dreams

As previously indicated, unless a neurophysiologic dysfunction is involved, everybody who sleeps has dreams. Hence the issue is related with not remembering the dreams. According to the Gestalt approach, one of the reasons for not remembering dreams is the fact that the person does not want to face with his/her personality characteristics he/she doesn't want to accept or own for various reasons (Perls 1969, 142). However, by ignoring those parts of our personality we do not like we cannot make them disappear. If we do not accept them, if we do not integrate them within our personality and if we do not take responsibility for them, these characteristics carry on their existence in a chaotic way, beyond our control, and they emerge at the most inappropriate times and in harmful ways, often leaving us in a difficult position.

Another reason for not remembering dreams is the fact that the person may not wish to realize his/her needs for whatever reason. Those who do not remember their dreams, remaining unaware of their needs, avoid the responsibility of changing the missing or erroneous aspects of their lives. However, this avoidance of responsibility makes them unhappy, more hopeless, and more anxious.

One other reason for not remembering dreams is the person's unwillingness to accept or to express to others the feelings that he/she finds negative or inappropriate. However, even though the person does not like it and tries to repress these feelings, they are there, and the failure to express them gives rise to unfinished business and a deterioration in relations.

For these reasons, Perls (1969, 247) suggests those clients who cannot remember their dreams to establish a dialogue with their dreams that starts with "Where are you, my dreams?" During this dialogue, by changing places, the client talks both as him/herself and also as the forgotten dreams; meanwhile, both parties express their thoughts and feelings to each other.

Below is an example of the work done with Allan, who had not been able to remember his dreams for years.

Allan:	*My dreams, where are you? Why don't you show yourselves to me?*
Allan (as his dreams):	*We show ourselves to you, but you don't want to remember us, whereas we have important clues for you.*
Allan:	*You are scaring me. What do you know about me that I don't?*
Allan (as his dreams):	*What are you afraid of discovering about yourself?*

Allan:	*I don't know! Do you have any idea?*
Allan (as dreams):	*You have a school problem which makes you unhappy and bothers you, could it be related to this?*
Allan:	*Yes, school bothers me, but what does it have to do with you? The cause of the school problem is the ridiculous education system, not me.*

As this dialogue progressed, Allan eventually started to realize his projections related to the school problem and how he avoided taking any responsibility for solving it. It is quite obvious that such dreamwork is a useful method in making a person realize what he/she is avoiding in terms of awareness and responsibility taking.

Remembered Dreams

Narrating the Dream

Dreamwork starts with narrating the dream. However, in the Gestalt approach, the dream needs to be told not as a past event but as if it is being experienced at that moment. For example, instead of narrating the dream as "I was sitting with my husband at a restaurant we frequently visited . . . the client is asked to tell his/her dream in the present tense as "I am sitting with my husband in a restaurant we frequently visit. A man in a plaid shirt comes to our table, and he asks something to my husband, but I cannot hear what he is asking". The purpose of this is to enable the person to adapt to the dream more quickly and to avoid regarding the dream as something unrelated to him/her and as a past experience (Fantz 1998, 54).

In the Gestalt approach, dreamwork can be carried out in many ways. Julie's dream will be given below to demonstrate aspects of how the work can be carried out.

Julie's Dream

I am sitting at the airport with my mother. I will be going abroad in a little while; my mother has come to see me off. While we talk, I suddenly realize that I don't have my ticket. When I tell this to my mother, she says that it might be in her purse, she opens it, and starts to rummage in her purse for my ticket. Then she says, "There! I've found it," but what she has found is not the ticket but my passport. I panic, rush around, and start asking everybody around, "Have you seen my ticket?" Finally I find the ticket in my mother's purse, but there is no destination or departure time written on it. That is, the ticket only has my name but no other information.

Giving a Voice and Playing Various Parts of a Dream

In the Gestalt approach, one of the methods that can be used during dreamwork is giving a voice and playing various parts of a dream. During such work, first of all, every person, object, situation, feeling, and the like included in the dream is defined, and then the dreamer talks about each as if he/she is the person, object, situation, or feeling in the dream in the form of "I" statements. While acting, the actor expresses everything about that person, situation, object, or feeling with his/her posture, body movements, voice, and facial expressions. At the core of this work lies the belief that everything we see in a dream is actually a part of ourselves. Hence, the goal is to be aware of all the projected parts of ourselves not only by talking—i.e., at an intellectual level—but also by experiencing and feeling it. In such work, priority should also be given to the setting of the dream, that is where the dream takes place. This gives an impression of the existential background (Perls 1969, 297). For example, the dream in the example above takes place in an airport. The meaning of the airport for Julie gives a general impression of how she sees herself and her way of being in her present life. Julie's first-person expressions of herself as the airport, as herself, as her mother, as her mother's purse, as the ticket, passport and the feeling of panic are given below.

As the airport in the dream: I am the airport. I am not very big, but passengers feel comfortable in me. They can find their way easily, I am not complicated. I am clean and orderly. Many people visit me. I help them to go somewhere, to some event, or to their loved ones. This makes me very pleased with myself.

As herself at the beginning of dream: *I am Julie. I am sitting at the airport with my mother. I frequently go out of town and abroad. It seems I am going on a business trip now. I am very happy that my mother has come to the airport to see me off. I wish she could come with me.*

As her mother in the dream: *I am Julie's mother. My daughter is going to a meeting abroad. I have come to the airport to see her off. I will miss her very much. She travels frequently. I am used to it, but I still miss her every time, and I am proud of her. I like seeing her off and welcoming her back.*

As the purse in the dream: *I am Julie's mother's purse. I am practical and strong. I have many things inside. Many things people may need. This really pleases me.*

As the passport in the dream: *I am a passport. I am Julie's passport. I know who Julie is. Julie cannot go abroad without me. I am helping her to learn new things, to see new places, and to get to know new people. I am contributing to her development, and I like that very much.*

As the ticket in the dream: *I am a ticket, but I am blank, that is, the destination they will use me for is unclear. Therefore I am useless. Actually I am both useful and useless. I could be very useful, but at the moment, I am completely useless. I am sorry.*

As the feeling of panic in the dream: *I am the feeling of panic. People don't like me at all. I make them unsure of what to do and unable to think. My color is dark gray, and I do not have a definite shape, so I can take any shape, go anywhere, and get people under my control. At the moment I am controlling Julie. She is confused and scared.*

Julie, while expressing herself verbally as the different parts of the dream, also acted out the parts. For example, when she was her mother, she sat like her mother, she talked in her style, and she rummaged in her purse as her mother does. When acting as herself, she sat and acted as she did in the dream and rushed around. When she became the purse, she acted through her body language as a very functional and strong bag with many things inside.

Julie had this dream six months after she lost her mother. After expressing and acting different parts of the dream, Julie realized that she was very happy to help people (the airport) and to be able to give them what they need (the purse), that she loved her mother very much, and she missed her (herself), that her mother also loved her, and was proud of her (her mother), that she liked to learn new things, and to see new places (the passport), but at the moment, after losing her mother, she did know where to go and what to do (the ticket), and because of that, she was in a state of panic, confused and scared.

In some dreams, the dreamer him/herself might not be involved. In terms of dreamwork, whether or not the person is in the dream makes no difference as everything in the dream is anyway reflects him or her. Sometimes, in such cases, the person might be asked to choose to be one of the people, objects, situations, and so on, as his/her starting point, and to narrate the dream from the point of view of whatever is chosen (Rebelliot 2004).

Perls (1969, 190) indicated that working on nightmares in particular is very useful in raising awareness of what is rejected and disowned—those parts of the personality thus projected—and in integrating these parts into the personality. However, for most people, it is very difficult to give a voice to and enact those horrible, bad, and ugly creatures or persons in their dreams because these are the parts that are the most alienated and the most rejected. For example, if a person dreams about a wild dog or a person he/she does not like at all, he/she may avoid and resist behaving like that dog or person, to assume their posture, or to sound or talk like them. In such situations, the client first might be asked to describe the creatures, animals, or people in the dream, to visualize them, and then to talk about their characteristics. For example, Marleen described the wild dog she dreamed about as being very strong; it can bite those it does not like, can harm them, and can protect itself. People are afraid of it and are cautious of it. They cannot harm it because it would not allow it. Despite the fact that in the beginning Marleen did not want to talk about the characteristics of this wild dog, once she started relating its characteristics, she saw the strength the dog had for self-protection and for stopping other people from harming it, and she realized that to possess such strength was not a bad thing after all. Upon realizing this, she was able to enact the wild dog and was willing to own this strength. From the Gestalt perspective, when a person integrates into his/her personality those characteristics previously ignored, nightmares stop because now the person has internalized his/her disowned characteristics and has become stronger (Mackewn 1996, 123).

Creating Dialogues among Different Elements of a Dream

In the Gestalt approach, another method that can be utilized in dreamwork is to create dialogues among different elements of the dream. This practice should always be carried out after giving voice to the elements and enacting them. In this practice, the person is asked to create dialogues among all the elements of a dream or among those he/she finds significant. During dialogue creation, double- or triple-chair techniques can be utilized. A dialogue may start from any scene of the dream according to the person's choice. An example of such a practice could be the dialogue Julie established with her mother during her dreamwork:

Julie: *Mother, I am going again. I am going to miss you all. Take good care of yourselves while I am away.*

Mother: *Don't worry about us. Go, and do what you must do. And rest a little; you tire yourself too much. What time does your plane leave?*

Julie: *I don't know exactly. Let me check. I don't have my ticket, where is it?*

Mother: *Hold on; don't worry, maybe it is in my purse.*

Julie: *I hope so; I always find what I am looking for in your purse. I hope it is there.*

Mother: *Aha! I think I got it. Noooo! It is the passport.*

Julie: *My God! What am I going to do? Where is my ticket?*

Mother: *Hold on, don't panic. We will find it. If the worst comes to the worst, we can purchase another ticket.*

Julie: *Take another look in your purse, maybe it slipped under something.*

Mother: *Yes, here it is. Take it.*

Julie: *Mother, you are always a lifesaver. Thank you so much. But this ticket has no destination; there is no flight number, no departure time. It only has my name.*

(At that moment, tears started to flow and the rest of the dialogue turned into Julie's expression of her feelings for her mother, who had passed away six months previously.)

Julie: *Mother I miss you so much. You went on a trip and left me behind. I don't know where you are, I don't know what you are doing. Life without you is so tough. I feel so alone. I don't know what to do, where to go, how to get there. I feel helpless and I have no energy. It is as if I got lost in life.*

Mother: *Honey, I would never want to leave you behind but you know how hard my life was over the past year. I could never enjoy anything. But I love you so much. You always supported me. I am proud that I have a daughter like you. But please don't let yourself go, remember who you are. You have kids; you have your job, your friends. Please don't lose your joy. You still have a lot to do. Even though I am not beside you physically, actually I am always with you. Please be strong and carry on. I am behind you in whatever you do. Actually you know well where you are going.*

Julie: *I am so lonely, I don't want to do anything. Life has no meaning. Nothing can take your place! I wish I could hug you just once more. Now I can understand better how lucky I was to have a mother like you. Sometimes we made each other mad, but I apologize for all those times.*

Mother: *No need for an apology. It was nothing. At times I acted foolishly too. But we always knew that we loved each other. If it weren't for you, I could not possibly endure certain things as you well know. Come on my lovely girl, pull yourself together and carry on for me. Have a safe journey. Come on . . .*

While working with Julie on her dream, another dialogue came up between herself and the blank ticket:

Ticket: *I am blank, I am a ticket, but I am useless. I cannot take anybody anywhere. I feel as if I am good for nothing.*

Julie: *Why don't you tell me where I should go? I must go somewhere; otherwise you wouldn't be in this dream. But where am I supposed to go? I feel lost.*

Ticket: *Where would you like to go?*

Julie: *Nowhere. But since you were in my mother's purse, she wants me to go somewhere. I suppose she wants me to carry on with my work abroad. I think she wants me to carry on with the last job I was involved with.*

Ticket: *Yes, the one in Germany. How would you feel if I had a Frankfurt destination?*

Julie: *But I don't want to go. What good will it serve? I feel so lonely, and that course has also lost its meaning, just like everything else.*

Ticket: *What else would you feel? Your mother wants you to go; look, she came to see you off and she gave you your passport.*

Julie: *I don't know, I honestly don't know. Maybe later, I am not ready yet. Does my mother really want this? But I still miss her very much.* (Here, Julie started to cry again.)

Dialogue experiments can serve many purposes. The dialogue in this example was oriented toward Julie's completing her unfinished business with her mother and her rearranging of her way of living. Dialogue work is also very helpful in solving an impasse, in recognition of needs, in changing the styles of contact, and in integration of the polarities.

Drawing the Picture of the Dream

During dreamwork, one other method that can be used is drawing a picture of the dream. In this practice, the person can be asked to draw the whole dream or a segment of it that is significant for him/her, the scariest part of the dream, or the feeling the dream evokes. Another approach could be to draw different parts of the dream on separate cards in sequence. Drawing can help the person to come closer to the meaning of the dream and to be more aware of his/her feelings (Mackewn 1996, 146).

Completing the Dream

One of the methods that can be used, particularly when working with unfinished dreams, is the completion of the dream by the client. During this work, the person is asked to visualize the seen part of the dream as if living it in the present moment and to complete it in any way he/she wants (Mackewn 1996, 144). Such work can be very useful in terms of reaching awareness of needs and in finding the ways to satisfy those needs. In some cases, while trying to complete the dream, people who were not in the original dream but who can provide support for the client can also be allowed to enter the dream. For example, during dream completion practice, Julie included her father in the dream. She visualized that her father also came to the airport while she was searching for the ticket with her mother and told her that she had left her ticket at home and he had brought it as soon as he noticed. Hence, on one hand, Julie's destination and time of departure was determined, and on the other hand, the meaning of her existence (e.g., carrying on with her work) was supported by her father. Carl Whitaker has indicated that another possible approach during dream completion work could be to include the therapist in the dream (referred to in Fantz 1998, 59). During such work, the therapist can help the client to support him/herself where he/she was stuck in the dream by asking questions such as "If I were in this dream, what would my role be—what would I be doing or saying?"

Expressing the Dream with the Body

Yet another method that can be used during dreamwork is the expression with body posture of different parts, objects, or people from the dream. Later, by connecting these postures to one another choreography of the dream can be created (Daş 2002). The dream dance thus created can be performed with a specific music the client chooses to clarify the meaning of the dream.

Finding the Message of the Dream

The ultimate goal of all dreamwork is to reveal the covert and secret meaning of the dream and to understand its message. Hence, at the end of the dreamwork, the client is asked to sum up in a few words the message given by the dream. For example, the existence message Julie found related to her dream was this: "I feel lonely, I am in panic, and I find life to be futile. In order to overcome this, I must move on as soon as possible, deal with my work in particular, and develop myself. That is also what my mother wants."

The role of the therapist during dreamwork is to bring the dialogue to a deeper and more emotional level from its more obvious and shallow status. Integration and reaching the message of existence can only be achieved at this deep and emotional level. Accordingly, in the Gestalt approach, it is believed that, unlike in some other approaches, the message of a dream cannot be reached with purely intellectual explanations and interpretations but only by "experiencing" the dream (Frantz 1998, 48). During dreamwork, the therapist takes into consideration the inner conflicts, opposing poles, unfinished business, styles of contact, and impasses of the client and aims to help the client to raise his/her awareness of them. With this aim in mind, the therapist does not allow the client to avoid experiencing difficult situations, negative feelings and characteristics. On the contrary, he/she encourages and supports the clients to become fully immersed in them and to experience them intensely. For example, during work carried out with Julie, she first experienced intensely all her negative feelings such as loneliness, desperation, futility, and her longing and bereavement for her mother. While experiencing these feelings, she was able to come out of her long lived "strong role" and, by integrating both with her feelings and her mother, became really strong and reached a new message of existence where she could continue her development.

Dreamwork can be carried out on an individual basis or in a group. Dreamwork carried out in a group benefits not only the dreamer but also those who play different roles in the dream as this increases their self-awareness and helps them to relate different elements of the dream to their own lives. Zinker (1971) suggested the dreams be enacted as drama in groups and indicated that active participation of the group members as opposed to being mere observers would increase the depth and intensity of the experience. In this approach, which Zinker calls "dreamwork as theatre," the stage can be arranged in different ways. For example, the dreamer can be the director of his/her own dream and cast the group members as different people, objects, or parts of the dream, or he/she can also take part in it and ask other members which roles they would like to play. Another alternative is having the therapist cast the different roles.

In conclusion, the dream is a film that explains us and our lives to ourselves and we are the author, director, players, spectator, setting, and even the critic of it. As we grasp the meaning of this film, we will be one step further on our journey to integration and closer to a healthier and happier existence. Along this journey, the Gestalt therapy approach offers a very strong perspective and a wide range of methods that cannot be found in any other therapy approach.

19

A CASE PRESENTATION

In this chapter, the story, the diagnosis, and the therapy process of a case treated with the Gestalt approach, are presented. With respect to the professional ethical rules and the principle of confidentiality, in order to prevent the recognition of the person, the name and certain characteristics have been changed. Hence, the person is referred to as Mary. There are several reasons for choosing this patient as an example. The first is the client's being diagnosed as histrionic personality disorder according to the DSM-IV (APA, American Psychological Association, 1994) diagnostic criteria. Histrionic personality disorder is within the cluster B of Axis II diagnoses in DSM-IV. Among the psychiatric disorders, personality disorders are the ones that respond to therapy late. Moreover, among the personality disorders; histrionic personality disorder, antisocial personality disorder, borderline personality disorder, and narcissistic personality disorder, that are located within cluster B, are the hardest to treat. Furthermore, there are no drugs specific to these disorders. Generally, various drugs are prescribed according to the symptoms of the client. However, these are not therapeutic but rather they are used to suppress the symptoms. The second reason for choosing this case is that depression also accompanied the histrionic personality disorder as an Axis I diagnosis and the client twice attempted to commit suicide. Because of this, it was necessary to be more sensitive and attentive to the process of the client in therapy. Another reason is that the client had very annoying physical complaints such as fainting spells and distortion of her jaw that were adversely affecting her daily life. The most important factor determining the achievement of positive results in the treatment of personality disorders is the therapeutic relationship. However, particularly in cases of cluster B personality disorders, establishing and maintaining such a therapeutic relationship is not easy at all. While working with Mary, in addition to the difficulties associated with histrionic personality disorder, Mary's extreme pressure on me to "cure" these fainting spells and jaw distortions and her frequent anger with me for not being able to cure them immediately made the establishment and maintenance of the therapeutic relation even harder. The fourth and last reason for choosing this case is that even though Mary had previously used various medicines and had therapeutic help from time to time, there was no discernible improvement regarding her complaints.

The Case

Mary was twenty-six years old when she applied for therapy. She was a high school graduate, working in the public sector and living alone.

Complaints

Her main complaints were serious problems in interpersonal relations, lack of self-confidence, distortion of the jaw, fainting spells, difficulty in concentrating, a lack of interest in life, feelings of loneliness, and lack of appetite.

Initial Observation

Mary looked much younger than her age and she was pint-sized. Her very short hair and thinness stood out. During the first interview, she was having a very sad facial expression and cried from time to time. She was talking slowly and in a rather low tone of voice. She frequently used the expression "nobody can help me." She looked down and avoided eye contact while talking. Nevertheless, she showed an effort to answer the questions.

The Story

Mary was born in a small town with the help of a midwife at the expected time and in the normal way. She was the eldest of a family with three children. Her father was a high school graduate, while her mother had only finished elementary school. Mary has a sister two years younger and a brother four years younger. Because of her father's job, the family moved frequently to different places, and Mary lived in various towns and cities until she was twelve.

Because of her father's heavy drinking problem, there were violent fights at home. During these fights her father sometimes beat her mother, and from time to time, Mary, as being the eldest child, was also beaten. During these fights, the mother usually ran away from home with her youngest child and did not come back for several days. Thus, Mary occasionally had to take care of her sister till she was eight years old. Her father used to come home late after drinking with his friends, and on those nights, Mary was scared to stay alone with her little sister at home. Mary explained her feelings like this: "I didn't know which one was scarier: staying at home alone with my little sister or waiting for my father without knowing what would happen when he came home drunk." Anything could be a reason for the fights, but the main reasons were her father's jealousy of her mother and his insulting her. Sometimes, when her father got very angry, he threatened to kill them all with a knife. Her mother was also very short tempered. Whenever she was angry at her husband, she used to take her anger out on her children and treat them badly. She beat Mary and her other daughter the most but didn't beat her son much, either because of his being a boy or being young. Eventually, when Mary was thirteen years old, her mother left home and did not come back for three or four months. During these months, her father started to sexually abuse Mary. Mary was very afraid of him, and not knowing what to do, she was crying continuously. Her distressed mood attracted the attention of her teacher at school, and she called her father to talk about Mary, but he did not go to meet her. As the father did not show up, the teacher wrote a letter to her mother. After receiving the letter, her mother came back home, and they started to live together again. The father still continued to abuse her, and sometimes her sister as well. Then Mary decided to tell her mother about her father's sexual abuse. Her mother did not believe her, accused her of lying, and kicked her out. As Mary didn't have a place to go, she went to her teacher's home. When she told her teacher about what had happened at home, the teacher decided to talk with her mother the next day. As a result of this conversation, the mother became convinced that Mary was not lying, and they returned home together. That night there was a huge fight at home, and the father kicked his wife and all the children out of the house. They first went to the house of her aunt who was living in a nearby town and later to the grandmother's home. Meanwhile her parents were divorced. The grandmother was economically very poor and soon started to complain of the added burden. The mother was fed up with these complaints and felt compelled to marry a man with two children of his own within two months. In the beginning, the stepfather treated Mary and her siblings decently, but in time, he started both fighting with her mother and mistreating the children. He did not have an alcohol problem, but he had a habit of making obscene remarks and nicknaming the girls with bad words related to their bodies.

Mary's school performance was generally either average or slightly above average. She was an introverted, quiet student who avoided causing any trouble. She was determined to run away from home as soon as she finished high school but she did not share this with anybody. Actually, as soon as she graduated, she went to stay with a relative who was living in another city. She stayed there for a while, helping with the housework and caring for the children, but when they had to move to another city, she started to look for a job. Eventually, she started to work in a company on the recommendation of her relative. As she was earning a very low wage, she could only afford to rent a very cheap house in poor condition and confined herself to eating one meal each day that was provided by the company. During this period, her sister couldn't bear the situation at home any longer and came to live with her. At about the same time, Mary started to have an affair with one of her bosses at work. She wasn't happy at all with this relationship, but she carried on as she was scared to be fired from work. However, later she became pregnant, and when this was learned, she was fired anyway. In the meantime, her sister had left home and started to live with her boyfriend. Her sister's boyfriend was a good person and found a new job for Mary.

Although Mary did not like this new job and frequently had problems with her superiors, she tried to endure the job because of its advantages. However, one day, she had a very bad quarrel with one of her bosses and fainted for the first time in her life. During this spell, which lasted about fifteen minutes, she could hear the sounds around her although not very clearly but could not move a single muscle no matter how she tried. After this, whenever she became very angry or sad, she started to faint. In time, the people at work started to make fun of her situation. They even made cutting remarks like "Don't say anything to her, she will faint." On one occasion, she was so bothered by such a remark that her lower jaw was distorted toward the left, and she could not talk. Afterward, whenever she was extremely sad or stressed, the same thing repeated. The distortion of the jaw sometimes lasted for three or four minutes and sometimes as long as ten to fifteen minutes. She went to see a psychiatrist a few times because of the fainting spells and jaw distortion and attended therapy from time to time, though not on a regular basis. The drugs that were prescribed reduced the number of fainting spells and jaw distortions but failed to cure them permanently. She started to become more and more hopeless, taking no pleasure from life and having difficulty in sleeping. She was feeling desperately alone, and in order to assuage this loneliness, she would go out and have one-night stands. Mary justified these experiences thus: "At least, I wasn't feeling lonely and hopeless for a few hours." However, when her partners did not call her again in the following days, she felt worse.

Mary eventually had a long-term relationship. She loved him very much and thought that he loved her too. However, three months later, they started to abuse each other physically, and they broke up. In those days, her mother divorced her second husband and moved in with her. Mary initially welcomed this new situation as she would not be alone any longer, but they started to argue after a while. One day, they argued so badly that Mary felt distraught and attempted suicide by swallowing pills. Mary explained the reason for this suicide attempt like this: "I wanted to punish my mother; but also, I could not find a reason to live any longer." However, as she had left the boxes of the pills she took in their living room, after a while, her mother found them, realized what had happened, and took her to the hospital. But as her mother was still very angry with her because of the fight, on the way to the hospital, she said several times, "I hope you will die," and hearing these words saddened Mary further. After the initial treatment, Mary was suggested to be put on the waiting list for admission to the psychiatric ward, but she flatly refused this. After a short while, her sister also broke up with her boyfriend and came to live with them. As her mother always favored her sister, Mary felt left out most of the time. Since neither the mother nor the sister was working, Mary was the sole breadwinner of the house, but still she couldn't endear herself to them. The three of them fought often. During this period, the fainting spells and distortion of the jaw continued, though not as frequently as before.

One day, they had such a big fight at home that the neighbors had to call the police, and they were taken to the police station. Mary met a policeman there, and they fell in love with each other. Their relationship went very well for about four months. Mary, very much in love, was trying to do whatever he wanted. She even paid off all his debts. Their only problem was not being able to see each other more often and for longer. Whenever Mary asked about the reasons for this, her boyfriend did not give a clear answer and fudged the question, answering just with, "I am busy." This answer bothered and frustrated her a lot and even led to fights from time to time. Later, when Mary became pregnant, he confessed that he was married. Then Mary attempted to commit suicide for the second time. After taking a cocktail of all the pills that she could find at home, she went to a nearby park and lay down on a bench. A person who saw her sleeping there saved her life by calling the police. This time, she was in a really bad condition, and as she did not want to return home, she accepted the offer of hospitalization. Mary explained her feelings and thoughts on those days like this: "I reevaluated my life when I was in hospital and became fully convinced that I had two paths ahead. I would either say, 'It isn't worth living,' and decide to leave this world for real, or I would say, 'It is worth living,' and decide to stand on my own feet despite everything. I was so tired and hopeless that I had almost deciding to quit, but when I saw the efforts of the doctors to understand me, I started to say, 'Maybe it is worth living,' and I decided to try."

I met Mary two months after she got out of the hospital. The psychiatrist who was responsible for her treatment in the hospital called me and gave me some information about her. Later Mary made an appointment, and after the initial evaluation session, she decided to start therapy. We met regularly once a week for ten months, once every ten days for the following thirteen months, once every two weeks for the following year, and once a month for another year.

Gestalt Diagnosis

There is no doubt that diagnosis is the basis of treatment. In the Gestalt approach, which builds upon existentialist, phenomenological, and holistic viewpoints, diagnosis is made using various maps focusing on different characteristics of the person-environment interaction. There are various maps that can be used in diagnosis. Which map or maps are going to be used is determined according to the preference and knowledge of the therapist. In the following pages, the maps that were used in the diagnosis of this particular case and the characteristics of the case in terms of these maps are given in detail.

The maps used in diagnosis were

a. capacity for contact
b. the feelings of the therapist
c. completion of the need cycle
d. contact styles
e. the rhythm of relation
f. support systems

These maps, right from the beginning of the therapy, start to inform the therapist about the path to be followed, but during the whole therapy process, it might be necessary to readjust the maps according to new observations, information, and developments.

THE MAPS

a. Capacity for Contact

In the Gestalt approach, one of the maps that can be used in the evaluation of the client is related to his or her "contact ability." Yontef

(1993, 415) stated the most determining characteristics of the capacity to establish contact as the ability to show empathy, to establish intimate relations, to establish dialogue, and to express anger and joy.

Showing Empathy

Empathy means being able to understand the feelings, points of views, and the needs of others and to see the world through their eyes. During the evaluation, an effort is shown to determine with whom or under which circumstances the client can or cannot establish empathy. Lack of empathy is an indication of a very thick contact boundary. When evaluated from this angle, it can be said that Mary did not have the ability to show empathy to most of the people around her in recent years. For example, her immediate anger when her wishes and needs are obstructed, her continuous reproaches when her friends fail to contact her, or her failure to grasp the fact that she should not call her boyfriend four or five times a day are indicators that show that she has difficulty in showing empathy. On the other hand, in her childhood, when her mother left home and she had to take care of her brother and sister, her efforts to soothe her crying siblings and even her efforts to create toys for them from different materials show that as a child she had the capacity to empathize.

Establishing Intimate Relationships

Establishing intimate relations includes characteristics such as ability of a person to express him/herself for a long period of time without fear and with sincerity, ability to accept others without trying to change or putting pressure on them. From this point, it can be said that Mary cannot establish intimate relations in general and is mostly able to make only superficial contacts.

Even though it seems as if she had rather closer relations with her two boyfriends, these were not long lived. Mary, in general, confused intimate relations with sexual relations, felt very close even to people she had just met, and had sex with right away. On the other hand, when these people did not seek her out again or failed to do what she wanted, she would get extremely angry and send them away with furious and vicious outbursts. In her relations with her mother, sister, and a few girl friends she had, instead of sharing her experiences, she would compete with them, and at the end of such a competition, she humiliated either them or herself in an exaggerated manner. Throughout her life, the closest relation she ever established was the one with her teacher.

Establishing Dialogue

Dialogue includes characteristics such as explaining one's point of view and listening to others' viewpoints, negotiating to come to an agreement, struggling to reach goals, sustaining a relationship even when it is hard or disappointing and stepping back, giving up or letting go when necessary. From this perspective, it is seen that Mary with her "they would not listen or they could not understand anyway" attitude was avoiding having to express herself right from the beginning of her relations and was accepting the viewpoints of others immediately. An example of this can be her obediently doing whatever her boyfriends requested, especially at the beginning of her relations with them. In her relations, when her demands were not met and when she was disappointed, she could never tolerate the situation, and instead of negotiating, she would force the other party into submission. Whenever she felt that she was not receiving sufficient attention, she would display exaggerated manners, would not withdraw from the relationship, and would try to stay in the relation until she was harshly rejected. Despite all this, particularly after the third month of the therapy, Mary started to establish a good dialogue relation with me.

Expressing Anger

The dimension of expressing anger includes characteristics such as how the anger is expressed, and in expressing that anger, whether or not aggression is displayed, whether harm to others is taken into account, and whether an effort to control anger is shown. Mary, in general, showed her anger very easily and very quickly. While she generally expressed her anger verbally, there were times that she was physically violent. In other instances, she tried to keep down her anger, but after a while, it erupted uncontrollably. When she was angry, she was not able to take the possible consequences into consideration and could damage objects,

PROFF. DR. CEYLAN DAS

physically abuse her mother and sister, or by retroflecting her anger, could attempt suicide.

Expressing Joy

In this dimension, characteristics such as the expression of happiness, the situations where the person feels joyful, forms of entertainment that the person enjoys, and the topics that give the person pleasure are considered. Mary could express her happiness easily and again in an exaggerated manner. When she was in a good mood, she talked and laughed loudly. Dancing and drawing were among her hobbies. She enjoyed being with men, and even if she did not reach a climax, she saw sexuality as a form of entertainment.

b. Feelings of the Therapist

Another map that can be used in the evaluation of the client is the feelings of the therapist during the first few sessions. The basic idea behind this map is the belief that the client's mode of establishing a relation with his/her therapist and what the therapist feels about this mode of contact will be similar to his/her mode of establishing relations with other people around him/her and the feelings evoked in the others due to this relationship. The therapist, considering his/her her own feelings, can have the opportunity to obtain information about the contact styles that the client uses in his/her daily life and also to find the necessary clues that are needed to establish a satisfactory therapeutic relationship with the client (Yontef 1993, 411). Actually, in the Gestalt approach, the therapist uses him/herself as a tool in establishing a dialogic relationship with the client, not only during the first sessions, but throughout the whole therapy process. There is no doubt that, as therapy progresses and as the client changes, the feelings of the therapist will also change.

During the initial sessions, Mary felt the need to talk about how she was behaving correctly, how everybody was mistreating her, and how nobody understood her. It was very difficult for her to focus on the here and now. Our communication was mostly a monologue rather than a dialogue. The feeling of sadness was generally dominant. She talked slowly, her eyes staring right through me, her voice was very low, and sometimes it seemed as if she was talking to herself. Despite her sad tone of voice, facial expression, and even her tears, sometimes, all of a sudden and at an unexpected moment, she would ask in a loud voice for a cup of tea and then continue talking in a neutral tone. While listening to her, I could understand that, actually, nobody had listened to her carefully so far, and the best way of establishing contact with her would be just by listening to her. Very often, she evoked in me a desire to protect her. On the other hand, our sessions made me nervous because she was constantly checking and almost testing me to see whether or not I was listening to her properly and asking questions as if she wanted to undermine me. At the end of every session, she would ask, in a disappointed tone of voice, if I could help her and push me to give her a frame of time for when she would get well. She was expecting me to guarantee a solution to her problems and to regulate her relations, and as this was not possible, she became very angry, declaring that nobody cared for her, including me. In particular, she talked in a very exaggerated manner (by getting up, talking louder, and moving her hands and arms up and down) about her anger toward her colleagues at work or men, and while talking about these subjects, she would watch my face, check my reactions, and seemed to enjoy relating the injustices she experienced. Periodically, she would challenge me, asking, "They don't do such things to you, do they?" with a cynical expression. When she was not challenging, she would start pitying herself or trying to make me pity her with expressions such as "You obviously have not experienced such things, how could you possibly understand?" At such times, I really felt sorry for her and could understand that she had never taken the genuine attention of anybody. In either case, whether she was expressing either her sorrow or her anger, her exaggerated, superficial, and cynical attitude would make it extremely difficult to have good contact with her.

c. Completion of the Need-Satisfaction Cycle

In the Gestalt approach, the need-satisfaction cycle is another map that can be used when making a diagnosis. Life is an active cycle that goes on with the emergence of needs, the satisfaction of these needs, the establishment of the homeostatic balance, and the emergence of certain other needs (Simkin and Yontef 1984). The individual meets his/her various needs in the short or long term through this cycle. On the other hand, if a person experiences frequent interruption at various stages of this cycle and consequently fails to meet his/her needs, then the interaction between person and environment is disrupted and psychological problems emerge (Clarkson and Mackewn 1993, 69). Detailed information regarding the need cycle is given in the "Needs" section.

The individual has to possess the skills and abilities that would enable her to pass through each stage in order to complete this cycle. The earlier the stage of the cycle where the obstructions are experienced, the more rigid, fixed, and unchanging behavior characteristics that comes out (Clarkson 1993). At the same time, it can be said that when the interruptions are experienced at an earlier stage, the behavioral characteristics are (a) established at early ages, b) have a more physiological basis, (c) are less observable, and (d) are less suitable for therapeutic change. To produce a map that shows at what stage or between which stages the individual's need cycle was interrupted will help in determining the therapeutic interventions and strategies to be applied during the therapy (Keats 1996).

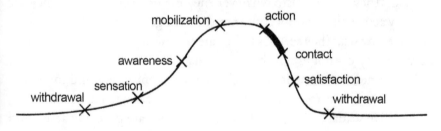

The need-satisfaction cycle of Mary shown as a wave

As can be seen in the above figure, when evaluated in terms of the completion of the need cycle map, Mary was interrupted between the action and contact stages of the need cycle. For instance, Mary was aware of her needs, such as to be loved, to be taken into consideration, to be appreciated. In order to meet these needs, she could take action and establish contact with people; however, either by approaching people who could not meet her needs or by acting inappropriately, she could not establish healthy contacts. To give an example, although Mary wanted to be appreciated at work, by lecturing people constantly, insisting on wearing miniskirts even though it was not permitted, and by behaving badly toward her superiors, she was not able to satisfy her need. In another instance, although she wanted to be loved by her sister and to have a good relationship with her, by throwing her out of the house from time to time, always buying her red clothes as presents even though she knew that her sister hated to wear anything red, or by leaving her in awkward situations, particularly in the presence of her boyfriend, she again was unable to meet her need. Similarly, by calling her boyfriend five or six times a day, by swearing uncontrollably when she was angry with him, and sometimes by insulting him sexually, she drove him away and failed to find the love and attention she needed. Thus, because she was not able to establish satisfactory contacts, she could not pass on to the next stages of the cycle such as satisfaction and withdrawal and cannot complete the need satisfaction cycle.

According to Zinker (1977, 108), persons who are interrupted between the action and contact stages are "hysteric" clinically. Such individuals talk a lot, do a lot, but cannot assimilate their life experiences. They are not aware of what they do and the consequences of their behavior. They have great difficulty in focusing their energy on a specific subject or field. They cannot taste whatever they eat or drink. Even if they are sexually active, they cannot concentrate on the genital sensations and thus do not enjoy sex. They seem as if they are not aware of their inner realities. Because they cannot establish good contact with others, they frequently feel emptiness and loneliness. Such feelings of emptiness and loneliness cause anxiety, and to compensate for this, overeating, substance abuse, or excessive sexual activity can be observed. They are generally active and their emotional state shifts frequently. Being the focus of attention is very important for them, and hence, they continuously focus on others but are only superficially interested in the thoughts and feeling of these others. They do well in short-term relationships but have great difficulty when it comes to establishing long-term and deep relations. They do not pay much attention to cognitive processes.

d. Contact Styles

In the Gestalt approach, one of the most important aims is to become aware of the contact styles that inhibit the individual's ability to establish healthy contact between him/herself and the environment and how to change them. For healthy contact, the boundary between the person and the environment should be both flexible enough to allow contact and yet rigid enough to allow each to remain unique (Simkin and Yontef 1984). When these boundaries are not sufficiently flexible or rigid, it leads to contact disturbances such as introjection, desensitization, projection, retroflection, deflection, egotism, and confluence. Information about each contact style was given in detail in the chapters called introjection, desensitization, projection, retroflection, deflection, egotism, and confluence. Below is a summary of the map of contact styles as it applies to Mary.

Introjection

Introjections are the information related to how the person perceives the world, how he/she sees herself and others. In particular, they are learned in childhood, but they are not assimilated. During the sessions with Mary, it was seen that the following introjections played a significant role in preventing her from establishing healthy contacts: Mary's life story is full of many dramatic events. The domestic violence she and the family had to endure due to her father's drinking problem, the mother's episodes of leaving home and abandoning Mary, her being forced to care for her siblings while she was in need of care herself, her mother's refusal to believe in her, and throwing her out while accusing her of being a liar have inevitably made Mary believe that she was "worthless and unimportant." Mary's sexual experiences started when she was very young with her father's abuses, continued with the obscene remarks of her stepfather and his verbal abuse regarding her body, and became worse with the affair she had with her first boss in early stages of her youth that ended with her pregnancy for which she paid dearly. All this led Mary to believe that men are bad and they seek only sex. Her mother was frequently beaten by her father and the only solution the mother could find was running away from home and leaving the children behind. Subsequently, her mother made an obligatory marriage for social and economic reasons, and she always had to live in very difficult and poor conditions. Observing her mother's disastrous experiences led Mary to believe that women are weak, and, so is she. Consequently, with all these beliefs in her mind, Mary came to the conclusion that "no relationship is safe," "I always have to be alert against the dangers that can come from other people," and "I should hurt in order not to be hurt."

Desensitization

The individuals that use desensitization as a contact style are unaware of their bodily needs and feelings and also unaware of the environmental conditions and the feelings and needs of others. Mary uses the desensitization style of contact very frequently. For example, her frequently forgetting to eat, staying up late even when she is sleepy, her refusal to take precautions despite the high risk of various diseases from her sexual relations with different people, and her abortions are all indicators of her desensitization toward her own body. Also, her fainting spells are a means of desensitization that she uses to cope with feelings she is unable to handle. On the other hand, her getting very angry when others fail to do what she wants without considering their needs and feelings, and her not even thinking about the possible connections between her humiliating and insulting attitudes toward her boyfriends or her mother and their becoming estranged from her are other examples of desensitization.

Deflection

In deflection, the individual fails to introject the positive or negative messages coming from outside, either by not really hearing them or by pretending not to hear them. Engaging in only small-talk in her relations with other people, her lack of concentration during sexual acts, and insisting on doing things in spite of the indications of others that they do not like them are the examples of Mary's deflections. Furthermore, during the sessions, whenever something positive was said to her, she would either suddenly change the subject or, by overfocusing on details, would wander away from the subject. Especially during the initial stages of the therapy, she pretended as if she did not hear questions regarding her family and start to talk about something else, and sometimes she would ask a question but continue to talk without waiting for the answer.

Projection

A projecting person, by reflecting his/her characteristics, feelings, thoughts, and wishes onto other persons, objects, or situations around him/her behaves as if they have nothing to do with her. For example, Mary frequently complained that nobody cared about her but was not aware of the fact that she herself did not care about others. She said that the men were always after sex, but she couldn't see that she also had an inviting attitude by going to clubs alone at very late hours. She accused her mother of being too demanding despite the fact that she herself frequently called and demanded several things from her. She mentioned that everybody forced her to do what they wanted, but actually she was also forcing them and got very angry when they refused to do what she wanted.

Retroflection

Retroflection is doing to yourself what you expected from others do to you or doing to yourself what you wanted to do to others. Mary's fainting spells, jaw distortions, and suicide attempts can be considered as the retroflection of her desires to make the others to faint, distort their jaws, or kill them. On the other hand, Mary is constantly seeking attention and love but, when she cannot find these in those around her, fails to provide attention and love to herself; that is, she cannot retroflect her attention and love, and instead either accuses or forces others for not showing attention and love to her.

Egotism

In egotism, the individual seems to be constantly watching and checking him/herself from the outside. He/she is always involved with him/herself and is concerned only with his/her body and feelings. Like all other types of contact, egotism is also beneficial and even necessary when used in the correct place and at the correct time. However, Mary almost never uses this style of contact. She does not think much about how her behaviors are seen from the outside and what sort of impressions she leaves on others.

Confluence

Confluence means that the person has no personal boundaries, and he/she flows together with another person or with his/her environment without a sense of differentiation. Mary had an unceasing desire to hold the center stage and to get attention, and because of this, she presented herself in widely different and exaggerated ways than others. However, her efforts to be different from everybody else kept her from being confluent, but at the same time, her efforts to be "too" different from others resulted in her being left out. Mary, in her relations with her mother, sister, and girl friends seldom experienced a feeling of "us" and often mentioned that she felt as if she "belonged nowhere." Hence, the difficulties she experienced in her relations were not derived from confluence but not being able to be confluent with others. In her relations with men, she wanted to stay in a permanent state of confluence, and when the other party did not allow this, she would become very angry.

e. The Rhythm of Contact

This map is used to define the rhythm of establishing contact of an individual with people who are important in his/her life. It was developed by Bob and Rita Resnick and is based on a cycle that is similar to the need cycle (Hemming 1999). The Resnicks call this the "re-lation-ship" cycle. They suggested that "re" means "again," "lation" means "contact," and "ship" means "ability," and thus the meaning of the name of the cycle is "the ability to establish contact over and over again." The cycle includes the stages of withdrawal, contact, close relation, confluence, and isolation. People who have the ability to establish contact over and over again can pass through all these stages one by one. They do not skip any stage, nor do they spend more time in any one stage than the others. For others, that is, who skip one or several of these stages or who spent too little or too much time in any one of these stages, then the rhythm of contact is disrupted, and a healthy relationship cannot be established.

At the withdrawal stage, both persons are ready to establish contact. To give an example, in this stage, both parties are on the way to the predetermined meeting venue. The contact stage is when this couple meets and starts a conversation. During the close relation stage, they chat by listening to each other, by understanding each other and by showing tolerance to their differences. At the confluence stage, they understand each other fully; they share common subjects and experience a feeling of "us." Then comes the isolation stage, and each turns toward his or her personal needs. After a while, the cycle starts again with the withdrawal stage. This cycle, similar to the need satisfaction cycle, can be shown in either a circle or a wave form. The rhythm of establishing contact shown as a cycle is given below. The gray and black spots resemble two persons.

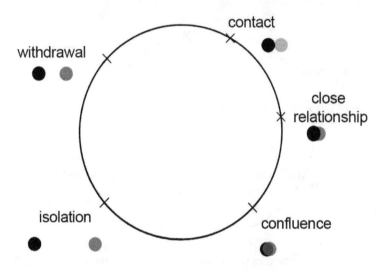

The rhythm of contact shown as a cycle

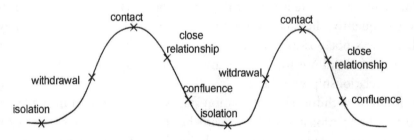

The rhythm of contact shown as a wave

If we look at the relations between Mary and the most important persons in her life, namely, her mother and her latest boyfriend, in terms of the rhythm of establishing contact, we can say that Mary had a healthy relationship with neither of them. In her relations with her mother, Mary remained in isolation for long periods of time, and sometimes, she did not speak to her for several weeks. When they saw each other, they would soon start fighting, and thus rapidly skipping the close relation and confluence stages, they would immediately pass into the isolation stage. The rhythm of contact of Mary with her mother is shown as a cycle below. As can be seen, the rhythm of the contact overly shortens the circuit between the isolation, withdrawal, and contact stages.

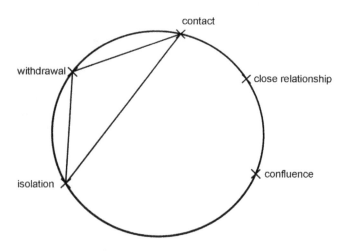

The rhythm of contact of Mary with her mother

Mary's rhythm of establishing contact cycle with her latest boyfriend was different than with her mother. Mary wanted to see him very frequently; she called him four or five times a day although she knew that it was not possible for him to answer it. She tried to meet all his requests and did not want to do anything without him. In other words, in her relationship with her boyfriend, Mary did not want to waste any time at the withdrawal and isolation stages. As can be seen in the figure below, the relationship of Mary with her boyfriend overly shortens the circuit between the contact, close relationship, and confluence stages.

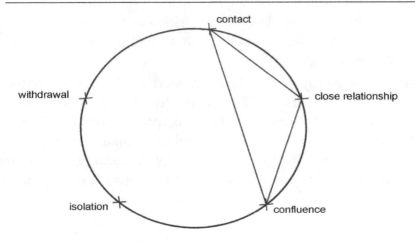

The rhythm of contact of Mary with her boyfriend

f. Support Systems

This map gives information about the person's capacity to support him/herself and use his/her environmental supports. The map consists of subdimensions, namely, interpersonal support systems, cognitive support systems, biological support systems, and the physical support systems in the environment (Mackewn 1999, 232).

Interpersonal support systems. To have an interpersonal support system means that there are people around the person with whom he/she has good relations and can share his/her problems and who like and protect him/her. In this respect, we can say that Mary's interpersonal support system is rather weak. Mary already has serious problems in her relations with people who are important for her. She also has problems at work, especially with her bosses, and does not get along well with her colleagues. She only has a better kind of relation with two sisters who live in the same apartment building and shares some of her troubles with them from time to time.

Cognitive support systems. Cognitive support consists of characteristics such as the intellectual capacity, educational level, speed of perception and the comprehension ability of a person. Mary's cognitive support systems are much better than her interpersonal support systems. The fact that she is a high school graduate and likes to read and the fact that she writes down the emerging significant issues after each session and elaborates on them are all positive points in terms of cognitive support.

Biological support systems. Biological support is related to the physical health of the person, his/her bodily characteristics, whether or not there is loss of an organ or its function, appetite, sleep conditions and the like. Even though Mary's physical health condition was generally good, her fainting spells, her difficulty in talking due to her jaw distortions, her loss of appetite, and the insomnia she experiences weaken her biological support systems from time to time.

Environmental support systems. The characteristics of the neighborhood and home, the available sporting and artistic activities, recreation and leisure venues, along with economic conditions can be considered among the environmental support systems. Mary was generally satisfied with the conditions of her neighborhood and her home. However, as her economic means were limited, she could not participate sufficiently in cultural and sporting activities, and the venues she had to choose for recreation and leisure were such mundane places that Mary actually did not enjoy visiting them. Consequently, as she has to spend most of her free time at home, it can be said that her physical environment is not very supportive.

Many contemporary Gestalt therapists believe that, in the evaluation of a case, it is not sufficient to use only Gestalt maps: it is also necessary for the therapists to be able to make a diagnosis according to the psychiatric classifications and also to have the skills to use various scales and projective tests that can be helpful in diagnosis. In this respect, for example, Delilse (1991), Greenberg (1989), Clarkson (1993), Shub (1998c), and Yontef (1988) have provided significant information about which therapeutic interventions would be beneficial and which interventions should be avoided, particularly for cases of personality disorders of cluster B, using Gestalt maps and DSM-IV or DSM-IV-R diagnostic criteria simultaneously.

DSM-IV Diagnosis

Mary's primary diagnosis, according to the DSM-IV (1994) classification, is histrionic personality disorder. The diagnostic criteria for histrionic personality disorder and the evaluation of Mary according to these criteria are given below.

Diagnostic Criteria for Histrionic Personality Disorder

A personality structure that is extremely sensitive and attention-seeking emerges in the early adulthood period and under different conditions as indicated by at least four of the following:

1. The person wants to be continuously trusted, admired, and praised.

2. The person's physical appearance and behaviors are inappropriately seductive.

3. The person has extreme interest in physical attractiveness.

4. The person shows his/her feelings in an inappropriate exaggerated style, e.g., passionately embracing persons he/she meets by coincidence, sobbing even in ordinary emotional situations, and experiencing outbursts of anger.

5. The person's feelings change suddenly, and he/she is superficial in expressing feelings.

6. The person becomes annoyed when he/she is not the focus of attention.

7. The person speaks in a style which provides only a general impression and which lacks details.

8. The person is egocentric; his/her actions are oriented toward immediate satisfaction; he/she cannot tolerate being prevented from achieving satisfaction.

When Mary's story and her attitude during the therapy are considered, it can be said that she complies with all of these criteria except the third one. The first criterion, which is about the desire to be continuously trusted, admired, and praised, has played a significant role in the deterioration of many of her relationships. For example, in her last relationship, Mary called her boyfriend four or five times a day, and when he could not take her calls because of his work, she would take this as a rejection and would start a fight that evening. This relationship lasted three months and ended in a very unpleasant way. Similarly, in her relations with her mother, even the mother's failure to thank her for buying the bread for dinner could lead to big quarrels. Mary's insistence on wearing miniskirts to work despite the fact that she was working in a very conservative environment or her overly inviting attitude toward the men she met at the clubs she visited are examples that can be given of the second criterion above. During the sessions, when Mary was talking about incidents, she would suddenly burst out in anger or she would exaggeratedly laugh or cry even when there was nothing really funny or sad. Furthermore, she could pass from one feeling to another very quickly in some sessions. That is to say, when she was crying she could start laughing immediately, and then in a very short time, she could become angry with something. This shows that Mary also complies with the fourth and fifth criteria. Fainting spells, suicide attempts, and an exaggerated way of talking and laughing were the ways Mary used to attract the attention of others when she did not receive sufficient interest. Although Mary wanted to be the center of attention at all times, her manner of talking about her experiences was extremely superficial. For example, the only information she gave about the boyfriend she claimed to be the reason for her second suicide attempt was limited to his being a police officer and that she loved him very much. She gave detailed information neither about his personality nor about his feelings, despite the specific questions asked about him. These characteristics of Mary comply with the sixth and seventh criteria.

Mary's habit of entering into sexual relations with men immediately and expressing her anger whenever she was angry regardless of the situation and conditions complies with the eighth criterion as an indication of her difficulty in postponing satisfaction.

In conclusion, it can be said that the primary diagnosis of Mary is histrionic personality disorder and this is accompanied by depression as an Axis I diagnosis. Although Mary was thinking that she had a good relationship with her latest boyfriend and was even surreptitiously making marriage plans, she was seriously traumatized when she found out that he was already married. Losing the meaning of her life and self-confidence, Mary came back from the critical border between life and death and, during the hospitalization following her second suicide attempt, decided to stand on her own two feet and to gain her self- confidence. Following the evaluations, it was seen that Mary's basic complaints were interpersonal relation problems and depression. It is thought that the difficulties she had experienced in terms of interpersonal relations were related to her histrionic personality disorder, so therapy was planned on that basis. Before going into the therapy process, it would be worthwhile to give some information about the point of view of the Gestalt therapy approach on personality disorders.

The Point of View of the Gestalt Therapy Approach to Personality Disorders

According to the Gestalt approach, character is the stylistic way an individual interacts with the environment (Shub 1999). It is the psychological signature of a person, and each person's signature is unique to him/herself. People, who have a personality disorder, always establish similar contacts depending on their core traits. In other words, those who have a personality disorder interact with their environment with the same rigid, fixed and static behavioral patterns. People with no personality disorder can behave in their relationships in a flexible, independent manner according to differing situations. For example, depending on the situation, they can give priority to themselves or others, can be very sensitive or relaxed, or can be very generous at times while tight-fisted in others. In other words, they have a wide repertoire of behavior and they can vary this repertoire as they wish. On the other hand, those with personality disorders cannot behave flexibly; on the contrary, they behave in the same way whatever the situations, conditions, or environmental expectations are. This restricts both their whole existence and their relationships.

The reasons for the emergence of personality disorders are childhood experiences. People with personality disorders have been exposed to very painful life situations over and over again. Such people have developed certain ways to survive and protect themselves in the face of painful experiences through creative adjustment. As the painful experiences were continuously repeated, they could not develop new styles of behavior as they grew up and as the conditions changed. In contrary, the styles of behavior they have developed in their childhood through creative adjustment became more rigid and fixed in time. As a result of this, they are able to adapt only in manners depending on which personality characteristics they developed.

The Goals of Therapy and Issues to Be Considered in the Therapy of Personality Disorders

In the Gestalt approach, the goal of the therapy of personality disorders is to make these fixed, rigid, and static behavior patterns flexible (Shub 1994b, 6). In other words, the goal of therapy is not to change the personality or to create a new one but the integration of the personality. In this way, it will be possible for the person to own the personality characteristics formally ignored, to be able to develop new alternatives under different situations, and to expand his/her behavioral repertoire.

According to the Gestalt approach, the success of therapy primarily depends on the therapeutic relation to be established with the client. However, while working with personality disorders, the establishment of a therapeutic relation is difficult and takes a long time. As previously mentioned, in histrionic personality disorder, the interruption is between the action and contact stages of the need satisfaction cycle. Hence, the contact skills of a person with histrionic personality disorder are severely impaired. Such individuals either establish contact in a much exaggerated way or not at all. Because of this, during therapy, the client should be allowed to express him/herself to the greatest extent possible and to experience emotional release. During therapy, no haste should be shown in applying Gestalt techniques except dialogic relation, and in the beginning, even efforts to increase awareness should be avoided. What is important is to make the client feel that he/she is being understood and accepted. While working with histrionic personality disorder, the therapist should be patient, calm, investigating, and participating but, particularly at the beginning, should be cautious in being directive, creative, or a catalyzer (see characteristics of the therapist). As such clients are mostly involved with their internal processes during contact, and as they frequently use desensitization, deflection, and projection as contact styles, they have great difficulty in the dialogic relation with the therapist. The therapist should never forget that histrionic personality characteristics are an outcome of creative adjustment made due to painful life experiences and should not refrain from putting him/herself forward no matter how disappointing his/her efforts to establish contact with the client are. However, if the therapist forces the client to establish a deep relation at the initial stage of therapy, when the client is not yet ready, then the therapeutic relation is disrupted, the client's interest in therapy diminishes, and he/she can terminate the therapy too early. For this reason, the dosage of contact should be very carefully adjusted.

As is the case with all personality disorders, clients with histrionic personality disorder are not aware of the rigidity of their behavior or how they establish contact with those around them. The therapist has to use the observations he/she made during the sessions very skillfully in order to help the client in becoming aware of his/her manners in establishing contact with the environment. However, while communicating his/her observations to the client, he/she should show great care; otherwise he/she may cause the client to feel guilty or embarrassed. In order to avoid this, the therapist should also explain to the patient about the viewpoint of the Gestalt approach on personality disorders, about creative adjustment, and about how his/her behavior has become rigid due to this creative adjustment. In particular, the fact that the problem is not a matter of the person being good or bad, but is caused by excessive rigidity of his/her personality, should be strongly underlined. As mentioned before, in cases of histrionic personality disorder, the clients are not aware of the impression they leave on others. Hence, one of the therapist's tasks is to give feedback regarding the impression that the client's behavior leaves on him/her. However, just as in communicating the observations, the therapist has to act with great care and should be ready for angry outbursts that may occur while feedback is being given.

Another issue to be focused on during therapy is to help the client to become aware of how limited his/her behavior repertoire is. While working on this repertoire, the self-harming behaviors of the client should also be pointed out. To this end, postponement of satisfaction, which is one of the most significant characteristics of histrionic personality disorder, should be particularly emphasized. On the other hand, clients with histrionic personality disorder have difficulty in abandoning this characteristic since slowing down, waiting, or procrastinating are extremely boring for them. They do not want to quit their exaggerated and enthusiastic style. This being the case, while working with persons with histrionic personality disorder, it is not easy for the therapist trying to reduce the energy level of the client on one hand, and trying to keep his/her interest keen in the environment and life in general on the other hand.

Therapy Process

To describe the therapy process in the Gestalt approach is very difficult, perhaps even impossible. Furthermore, as the treatment of personality disorders is a very long process with ups and downs, in order to grasp the process, it might be necessary to have each and every session described. However, as this is not possible, at this point, some sections of the therapy process will be described, and the most important points will be emphasized.

During therapy, Mary came to almost all sessions regularly. The first three months, in particular, were rather challenging. Mary's mood changed quickly, and she would generally give tough and negative reactions. Establishing contact with her was very difficult, and during the therapy, her most frequently used contact styles were deflection and desensitization. After explaining the meaning of deflection and desensitization and starting to work on how she could have learned these contact styles, Mary's attitudes during therapy began to change. When she became aware of how often she was using these contact styles in her daily life, she started to give examples she recognized and found great excitement in this. For Mary, the most difficult style of contact to accept and to recognize was projection. In particular, the session where she was complaining that "nobody cares about her feelings and wishes" was crucial as she became aware of the fact that she too did not care about the feelings and wishes of others. During the following three sessions, she experienced the anger and sorrow of this awareness. During this period, work was also carried out on the projections Mary made on her own body. The meaning of her fainting spells and jaw distortions were investigated. During these sessions, Mary realized how abusively she was treating her own body, how she did not care about her body or herself, how she was trying not to feel anything by holding her breath and by fainting, how her jaw distortions occurred when she felt vulnerable, and what she actually wanted was not to distort her own jaw but those of other people. In particular, regarding her relations with men, she became aware of how she needed to be confluent with them but, at the same time, because of her introjected message about "men are bad and seek only for sex" how she chose men who would not show her love and compassion, how she tried to attract men through sex alone, and how her not experiencing the love and warmth she craved could be the reasons for her failure to reach sexual satisfaction.

While working on needs, it became apparent that Mary did not pay any attention to her own needs for success and to be respected, and actually she did not believe that she could be successful and shown respect. Mary was not able to put her needs in order; she was always trying to meet her need for love and attention, and when she could not get the love and attention she wanted, instead of turning to other people, she kept pressuring the same persons who had already failed her. While working on these issues, Mary's unfinished business with her mother and father also entered the agenda. During sessions where two-chair and pillow practices were frequently used, Mary experienced very intense anger and sadness. Hence, at the end of the first year of the therapy, Mary's level of awareness regarding her needs, feelings, polarities, and styles of contact had considerably increased, her unfinished business with her mother and father had been investigated, and a satisfactory dialogue relation was established between us.

During this period, some changes also started to occur in Mary's life. For example, she was in a much closer relationship with the two sisters who were her neighbors; she bought a parrot and a cat and had not been entering into one-night stands during the past two months. She would visit her sister from time to time and manage not to fight with her. For Mary, the best improvements were her not having fainting spells or jaw distortions over the past five months. However, after a while, her mother divorced her third husband and came to live with Mary. She was not pleased with this, but as her mother did not have any other place to go and as she would have felt guilty if she had refused to let her stay, they started to live together. In the beginning, Mary was able to be more tolerant and could stop fights before they escalated. Although her mother was invited to the therapy sessions numerous times, she did not come to have a talk with me. In those days, Mary went for the first time on a three-day holiday with the two sisters with whom she was trying to have a closer relationship. Upon her return, she found that her mother had thrown her cat and parrot out, and this made her very upset.

They had a big fight that ended with her fainting. After this fight, Mary asked her mother to leave, and the mother moved in to her sister's house. The loss of the cat and the parrot, on one hand, and the latest fainting episode, on the other, led Mary to feel bad again, and the symptoms of depression reemerged. Her mother's throwing the parrot and the cat out triggered her own eviction memories and feelings related with this. While working on these, Mary's basic existential impasse which was on "to belong/not belong" theme, came out. She realized that in all her relations and in various fields of her life, she was living with this impasse. She had no friendships that had been sustained for years. After leaving home, at times, she lived with her mother and sister, but these periods did not last long. Although she had been working at the same institution for a long time, she had not established real contact with people there; she had mostly rebelled against the rules and frequently had problems with her superiors. In short, Mary embraced neither her work nor her relations and had not really committed herself to them. Another area where the effects of this impasse could be seen was her changing the houses she was staying frequently and without any reason and her leaving behind or throwing out most of her belongings when moving, even though her economic conditions were limited.

However, this impasse was most distinctively creating problems in her relations with men in two ways. First, Mary would enter into sexual relations with men and "belonged" to them in a sense, but as she did not commit herself to the relationship, she could not get sexual satisfaction. Secondly, Mary chose very short-term relationships during which she naturally did not feel any sense of "belonging," or she would go to the other extreme and in her long-term relationships she strive to "belong" excessively; however, as she was also afraid of "belonging", when her request was not fulfilled, she would become very angry and dismiss that person.

During our work related to this impasse, Mary realized that she was not feeling as if her body completely belonged to her. As this became apparent, the focus of therapy was shifted to body work, which led to the surfacing of the physical and sexual abuses in her childhood. She talked about these painful memories in such a superficial way and in such an emotionless tone of voice that it gave the impression that these things had not happened to her but to a character in a film or to someone else. When this was pointed out to her, she said that actually she did not want to talk about these things, and she had no feelings about these memories. However, these memories were experienced, and they would not disappear just because she did not want to remember them. Besides, these memories she wanted to forget formed the basis of her impasse. Because of this, even though it was very hard, she was asked to start a dialogue with her memories. This dialogue, which lasted almost two hours, started with "My memories, I don't want to remember you. How disgusting you are. You all look awful. Keep away from me. I erased you, don't you understand? You damned things!" During this dialogue, Mary lived out her sadness, her anger, and her shame in a most intense way.

In the following session, while we were talking about the "little Mary" who lived through all these events, her voice was very high pitched with a cynical tone. When this observation was shared with her, Mary said that she was irritated with the little Mary and only felt pity for her. These were very harrowing words, and in order to unravel the impasse, she had to make a good contact with little Mary and integrate with her. One of the ways that can be used in these instances is to work on photographs of the client. So I asked Mary to bring her childhood photographs to the next session, and her response was "I had very few anyway, and I tore them up." But when she came to the next session, she gave me an envelope, saying, "If you really want, you can put the torn pieces together." I opened the envelope, and when I saw the torn pieces of the photographs, I offered her to reassemble them together. She said,

"It is not worth it, don't bother, let us put them in the garbage." Putting them in the garbage was similar to putting little Mary in the garbage, so I refused and started to put the pieces together. She watched me putting the pieces together, and after a while, she joined me, and we managed to put together the majority of the pieces, if not all. However, the pictures were torn into such small pieces that even when put together, they did not mean much. At the end of the session, Mary left saying, "You can throw these out if you want." Later I put all pieces together and pasted them on separate pieces of drawing paper, and in our following sessions, she had very emotional dialogues with the little Mary in the photographs.

While working with the photographs, Mary would often come up with comments and questions such as "I don't look like anybody at home," "Do you think I resemble my father?" and "Do I look like my sister and brother?" When asked why this was important for her, her response was "No reason, I just asked." In the meanwhile, integration dialogues with the little Mary on the photographs were continuing, but when we came to the period of Mary's birth, she suddenly said, "Well, I am fine now, let us stop the therapy here." While talking about this sudden desire to stop, Mary stated that she had serious doubts about who her father was as her father often would point to her and ask her mother, "Whose child is she?" and her mother would never give an answer. She said that this unanswered question was worrying her very much and added that when she was little, in order to forget about this question, she used to sing loudly and dance. She also spoke in tears about how hard she had been trying to forget this subject for years. When I had asked her to bring her childhood photographs, she had been terribly afraid that the subject would come up, and she had decided not to say anything about it to me as she was terribly ashamed of this subject. In the following sessions, we started to work on this feeling of shame. In one of the sessions, Mary said that during her stay with her aunt she had found a photograph of herself when she was three months old, and she had it framed and hung it on the wall of her room. She also gave a copy of that photograph to me. Hence, Mary started to reconcile and integrate with her negative memories, her past, and herself.

During the following part of the therapy, we passed on to the expansion of Mary's behavior repertoire, and the intervals between the sessions gradually became longer and eventually the therapy came to an end. At that time, Mary had started a new relationship, which was progressing well. She got a new cat and parrot. Her relations at work were improving, and she had not fought with her superiors for some time. She called her mother and congratulated her on Mother's Day. She said that this was an indication of her acceptance of her "rebirth" and her forgiveness for her mother. She understood that she could not change her mother or the past but could accept them as they were. She was spending time with her sister's three-year-old daughter at weekends, and she was really taking good care of her. She said, "I love taking care of her during the weekends, because when I make her happy, it feels as if I am going back to my own childhood and meeting little Mary's needs." She joined a painting class and started to socialize with her course mates outside the class hours. One and a half years after the end of therapy, Mary brought an invitation card for an art exhibition. She was participating in an exhibition with other artists, and the picture on the invitation card was one of Mary's childhood photographs whose pieces I had put together and used in therapy. She had painted this photograph, and the name she gave to this painting was "rebirth." She neither fainted nor had jaw distortions again after the day when her mother threw out her cat and parrot.

REFERENCES

Aktaş, C. G. & Daş, C. (2002). Geştalt temas biçimleri yeniden düzenlenmiş formun Türk örnekleminde faktör yapısı, geçerliliği ve güvenirliği. *Temas: Geştalt Terapi Dergisi.* 1 (1), 81-108.

Amendt-Lyon, N. (2001). Art and creativity in Gestalt therapy. *Gestalt Review.* 5 (4), 1-31.

Baumgardner, P. & Perls, F. S. (1975). *Legacy from Fritz.* California: Science and Behavior Books.

Beisser, A. (1970). The paradoxical theory of change. J. Fagan & I. L. Shepherd (eds) *Gestalt Therapy Now.* New York: Harper & Row, 77-80.

Brown, J. (1998). *Back to the beanstalk: Enchantment and reality for couples.* Cambridge, Massachusetts: GIC Press.

Buber, M. (1958/1984). *I and Thou.* (2nd ed.). Edinburg: T & T Clark.

Burley, T. O. (1999). Reflections on insight and awareness. *GATLA Reader,* summer, 128-134.

Carlock, C. J., Glaus, K. H. & Shaw, C. A. (1992). The alcoholic: A Gestalt view. E. C. Nevis. (Eds.) In *Gestalt therapy: Perspectives and applications.* Mexico: The Gestalt Institute of Cleveland Press. 191-237.

Clarkson, P. (1991). *Gestalt counseling in action.* London: Sage Publications.

Clarkson, P. (1993 June 9-11). *The DSM-III R and Gestalt therapy workshop*. Metanoia. London.

Clarkson, P. & Mackewn, J. (1993). *Fritz Perls*. London: Sage Publications.

Clemens, M. C. (1997). *Getting beyond sobriety: Clinical approaches to long-term recovery*. San Francisco: Jossey-Bass Publishers.

Cohen, A. (2003). Gestalt therapy and post-traumatic stress disorder: The irony and challenge. *Gestalt Review*, 7, 42-55.

Crocker, S.F. (1981) Proflection. The Gestalt Journal IV (2, 13-34)

Crocker, S. F. (1999). *A well-lived life: Essays in Gestalt therapy*. NJ: The Analytic Press, Hillside.

Daş, C. (2002, march). *Rüya dansı* çalışma *grubu*. 4. ODTÜ Uluslar arası çağdaş dans günleri.

Daş, C. (2003 a) Geştalt ekolü öğretilerinin kişisel gelişime katkıları. (Ed.) A.E. Aslan. Örgütte *Kişisel Gelişim*. Ankara: Nobel Yayınevi.

Daş, C. (2003 b). Hangisi benim: İçe alınanlar. *Temas: Geştalt Terapi Dergisi*. 1 (2), 37-54.

Daş, C. (2004). Nefes al, ver ve harekete geç: Anksiyete ve Geştalt terapi yaklaşımı. *Temas: Geştalt Terapi Dergisi*. 1 (3), 127-140.

Delisle, G. (1991). A Gestalt perspective of personality disorders. *British Gestalt Journal*, 1(1):42-50.

Dement, W. C. (1960). The effect of dream deprivation. *Science*. 131, 1705-1707.

Downing, J. & Marmorstein, R. (1997). *Dreams and nightmares*. USA: Book Masters Inc.

DSM-IV (1994) *Mental bozuklukların tanısal ve sayımsal el kitabı*.. (Çev.) E. Köroğlu, Ankara: Hekimler Yayın Birliği.

Estrup, L. (2000). What is behind the empty chair? (Video cassette). Gestalt therapy, theory and methodology.

Evans, K. (1999). Brief and focal Gestalt therapy in a group. *British Gestalt Journal*. 8 (1), 24-36.

Fantz, R. E. (1998). *The dreamer and the dream: Essays and reflections on Gestalt therapy*. Cambridge: GISC Press.

Feder, B. & Ronall, R. (1994). *Beyond the hot seat: Gestalt approaches to group*. NY: The Gestalt Journal Press Inc.

Feder, B. (1994). Gestalt training in group. Bud Feder & Ruth Ronall (eds.) *Beyond the hot seat: Gestalt approaches to groups*. 167-179. New York: The Gestalt Journal, Press.

Fodor, I. E. (1998). Awareness and meaning-making: The dance of experience. *Gestalt Review.* 2 (1), 50-71.

Freud, S. (1915). *The handling of dream interpretation in Psychoanalysis.* London: Hogarth.

Freud, S. (1938/1966). *The basic writings of Sigmund Freud.* A. Brill. (Eds). New York: Modern Library.

Frew, J. E. (1997). A Gestalt therapy theory application to the practice of group leadership. *Gestalt Review.* 1 (2), 131-150.

Garcia, C., Baker, S., & DeMoya, R. (1999). Academic anxieties: A Gestalt approach. *Gestalt Review.* 3 (3), 239-250.

Goldstein, K. (1939). *The Organism.* New York: American Book Company.

Greenberg, L. S. (1979). Resolving splits: The two chair technique. *Psychotherapy: Theory, Research and Practice.* 16, 310-318.

Greenberg, E. (1989). Healing the borderline. *Gestalt Journal.* 12 (2), 11-55.

Harris, C. O. (1992). Gestalt work with psychotics. E. C. Nevis. (Eds.) In *Gestalt therapy: Perspectives and applications.* Mexico: The Gestalt Institute of Cleveland Press. 239-261.

Hemming, J. (1999, November 14-17). *Couple Therapy workshop.* Systemic Training Center. London.

Huckabay, M. A. (1992). An overview of the theory and practice of Gestalt group process. E. C. Nevis. (Eds.) In *Gestalt therapy: Perspectives and applications.* Mexico: The Gestalt Institute of Cleveland Press. 303-330.

Hycner, R. H. (1991). The I-thou relationship and Gestalt therapy. *Gestalt Journal.* 13 (1), 42-54.

Jacops, L. (1989). Dialogue in Gestalt theory and therapy. *The Gestalt Journal.* 12(1), 25-68.

Johnson, W. R. & Smith, E. W. (1997). Gestalt empty chair dialogue versus systematic desensitization in the treatment of a phobia. *Gestalt Review.* 1 (2), 150-162.

Joyce, P. & Sills, C. (2003). *Skills in Gestalt counseling and psychotherapy.* London: Sage Publications.

Jung, C. G. (1954/1968). Archetypes of the collective unconscious. H. Read, M. Fordham, G. Adler & W. McGuire (eds). *The collected works of C. G. Jung.* 9 (1), 3-41. London: Routledge and Kegan Paul.

Karon, B. (1976). The psychoanalytic treatment of schizophrenia. P. Magora (eds). *The construction of madness.* New York: Pergamon. 181-212.

Keats, A. (1996 28 November- 1 December). *Knowledge through process and DSM-IV workshop.* Metanoia, London.

Kempler, W. (1978). *Principles of Gestalt family therapy.* USA: The Kempler Institute Press.

Kepner, J. I. (1982). *Questionnaire measurement of personality styles from the theory of Gestalt therapy.* Unpublished dissertation thesis. Kent State University, Ohio.

Kepner, J. I. (1987). *Body process.* San Francisco: Josey-bass Publishers. Kepner, E. (1994). Gestalt group process. Bud Feder & Ruth Ronall (eds.). *Beyond the hot seat: Gestalt approaches to groups.* New York: The Gestalt Journal Press. 25-37.

Kitzler, R. (1994). The Gestalt group. Bud Feder & Ruth Ronall (eds.). *Beyond the hot seat: Gestalt approaches to groups.* New York: The Gestalt Journal, Press. 25-37.

Korb, M. P., Gorrell, J., & Van De Riet, V. (1989). *Gestalt therapy: Practice and theory.* Boston: Allyn & Bacon.

Köhler, W. (1947/1992). *Gestalt psychology.* New York: W.W. Norton & Company Ltd.

Latner, J. (1986). *The Gestalt therapy book.* New York: The Gestalt Journal Press, Inc.

Latner, J. (1992). The theory of Gestalt therapy. E. C. Nevis. (Eds.) In *Gestalt therapy: Perspectives and applications.* Mexico: The Gestalt Institute of Cleveland Press. 13-56.

Latner, J. (1995/1996). Reflections and memories: The contribution of Isadore From. *Studies in Gestalt Therapy*. 4-5, 63-84.

Lewin, K. (1952). *Field theory in social science: Selected theoretical papers.* London: W & R Chambers

Mackewn, J. (1996). *Modern Gestalt.* S. Palmeri, S. Dainow & P. Milner (eds). Counseling: The BAC counseling reader. London: Sage Publications.

Mackewn, J. (1999). *Developing Gestalt counseling.* London: Sage Publications.

McConville, M. (1995). *Adolescence: Psychotherapy and the emergent self.* USA: Jossey-Bass Inc., Publishers.

Mintz, E. E. (1994). The Gestalt therapy marathon. Bud Feder & Ruth Ronall (eds.). *Beyond the hot seat: Gestalt approaches to groups.* New York: The Gestalt Journal, Press. 116-133.

Naranjo, C. (1993). *Gestalt therapy: The attitude and practice of an atheoretical experientialism.* CA. Gateways/Idaho, Inc.

Nevis, E. C. (1998). *Organizational consulting: A Gestalt approach.* Cambridge, Massachusetts: GIC Press.

Nevis, E. C., Lancourt, J. & Vassallo, H. G. (1996). *Intentional revolutions: A seven-point strategy for transforming organizations.* San Francisco: Jossey-Bass Inc. Publishers.

Oaklander, V. (1992). Gestalt work with children. E. C. Nevis (eds). *Gestalt therapy: Perspectives and applications.* Mexico: The Gestalt Institute of Cleveland Press. 303-330.

Ornstein, R. E. (1972). The psychology of consciousness. San Francisco:W. H. Freeman.

Ovsiankina, M. (1928). Die wiederaufnahme von interbrochenen handlungen. *Psychologische Forschung.* 2, 302-389.

Özer, S. (2003). Fenomenolojimize açılan pencere. *Temas: Geştalt Terapi Dergisi.* 1 (1), 53-70.

Passons, W. R. (1975). *Gestalt approaches in counseling.* London: Sage Publications.

Perls, F. (1947/1992). *Ego, hunger and aggression.* New York: The Gestalt Journal Press.

Perls, F. (1948). Theory and technique of personality integration. *American Journal of Psychotherapy*. 2, 565-586.

Perls, F. (1969/1992). *In and out of the garbage pail.* New York: The Gestalt Journal Press.

Perls, F. (1969). *Gestalt therapy verbatim.* Lafayette, Calif: Real People Press.

Perls, F. (1973). *The Gestalt approach and eye witness to therapy.* USA: Science and Behavior Books.

Perls, F., Hefferline, R. F. & Goodman, P. (1951/1996). *Gestalt therapy: Excitement and growth in the human personality.* Great Britain: The Guernsey Press Co.

Perls, L. (1992). *Living at the boundary.* A Gestalt Journal Publication. Philippson, P. (2001). *Self in relation.* London: Karnac Books.

Philippson, P. (2002). *Uncertainty and choice.* http://www.gestalt.org/ Manchester Gestalt Center.

Polster, E. (1995). *A population of selves.* San Francisco: Jossey-Bass Publishers.

Polster, E. & Polster, M. (1974). *Gestalt therapy integrated: Contours of theory and practice. New York: Vintage Books.*

Rapp, E. (1994). Gestalt art therapy in groups. Bud Feder & Ruth Ronall (eds.) *Beyond the hot seat: Gestalt approaches to groups.* Brunner/ Mazel, Inc. 86-105.

Rebelliot, P. (2004 Autumn 20-28). *Advanced Gestalt training workshop.* Houkst, Frankfurt.

Reich, W. (1945/1972). *Character analysis.* New York: Simon & Schuster. Resnick, R. (1995). Principles, prisms and perspectives. Interviewed by Malcolm Parlett. *British Gestalt Journal.* 4, 3-13.

Rhyne, J. (1984). *The Gestalt art experience: Creative process and expressive therapy.* Chicago: Wadsworth Publishing Inc.

Ronall, R. (1994). Intensive Gestalt workshops: Experiences in community. Bud Feder & Ruth Ronall (eds.). *Beyond the hot seat: Gestalt approaches to groups.* New York: The Gestalt Journal, Press. 179-212.

Root, R. W. (1996). The Gestalt cycle of experience as a theoretical framework for conceptualizing the attention deficit disorder. *The Gestalt Journal*, XIX, 2 (fall). 9-50.

Rummel, R. C. (2004). *Psychological field theories: Understanding Conflict and War*. Vol I. The Dynamic Psychological Field. *www. hawaii.edu/power kils/dph.chap.3.htm.*

Schiller, C. (1994). *The little Zen companion*. New York: Workman Publishing Company.

Serok, S. (2000). *Innovative applications of Gestalt therapy*. Malabar: Krieger Publishing Company. 79-87.

Shapiro, C. M. & Flanigan, M. J. (1993). *Functions of sleep. ABC of sleep disorders*. C. M. Shapiro (ed). UK: BMJ Publishing Group.

Shepherd, I. (1970). Limitations and cautions in the Gestalt approach. J. Fagan & I. Shepherds (Eds.). *Gestalt therapy now*. Palo Alto: Science and Behavior Books.

Shub, F. S. (1994a). *Understanding awareness*. The working paper series. New York: A Publication of Gestalt Associates Press.

Shub, F. S. (1994b). *The process of character work: An introduction*. The working paper Series. New York: A Publication of Gestalt Associates Press.

Shub, N. F. (1998 a). *Wrestling the tiger: Working with introjections*. The Working Paper Series. New York: A Publication of Gestalt Associates Press.

Shub, N. F. (1998 b). *Gambling and Gestalt therapy workshop*. AAGT 3rd Annual International Gestalt Therapy Conference, 3-7 June. Cleveland, Ohio.

Shub, N. F. (1998 c). *A methodology of borderline treatment*. The Working Paper Series. New York: A Publication of Gestalt Associates Press.

Shub, N. F. (1999). Why Gestalt therapy is particularly helpful for treating character-disordered clients. *Gestalt Review*. 3 (1), 64-77.

Sills. C., Fish, S. & Lapworth, P. (1998). *Gestalt counseling*. Oxon: Winslow Press Limited.

Simkin, J. (1974). *Gestalt therapy*. Mini-lectures. Milbrae. CA: Celestial Arts.

Simkin, J. S. & Yontef, G. M. (1984). Gestalt therapy. R. J. Corsini (eds.). *Current Psychotherapies.* Illinois: F.E. Peacock Publishers. 279-320.

Smith, E. W. L. (1977). *The growing edge of Gestalt therapy.* New York: The Citadel Press.

Stern, D. N. (1985). *The interpersonal world of the Infant.* New York: Basic Books.

Tuğrul, C. (1998). *Female sexual dysfunctions and Gestalt therapy workshop.* AAGT 3ʳᵈ Annual International Gestalt Therapy Conference, 3-7 June. Cleveland, Ohio.

Tuğrul, C. (1999). *Shame, guilt and sexual dysfunctions workshop.* AAGT 4ᵗʰ Annual International Gestalt Therapy Conference, 26-30 May. New York.

Türkçe Sözlük (1995) Milli Eğitim Bakanlığı yayınları 2798: Ankara Tyler, D. M. (1994). Gestalt movement therapy in groups. B. Feder & R. Ronall (eds.). *Beyond the hot seat: Gestalt approaches to groups.* Brunner/Mazel, Inc. 105-116.

Wheeler, G. (1998). *Gestalt reconsidered: A new approach to contact and resistance.* Ohio: The Gestalt Institute of Cleveland Press.

Wheeler, G. & Backman, S. (1994). *On intimate ground: A gestalt approach to working with couples.* San Francisco: Jossey-Bass Inv., Publishers.

Wingfield, E. (1999). Performance anxiety in classical singers and musicians. *British Gestalt Journal.* 8 (2), 96-107.

Woldt, A. L. & Stein, S. A. (1997). Gestalt therapy with the elderly on the "Coming on Age" and completing Gestalts. *Gestalt Review.* 1 (2), 163-184.

Yolaç, P. & Tuğrul, C. (1991). *Vaginismus tedavisinde Geştalt yaklaşımı.* 27. Ulusal Psikiyatrik Bilimler Kongresi, 6-9 Kasım. Antalya, Türkiye.

Yontef, G. M. (1979). Gestalt therapy: Clinical phenomenology. *The Gestalt Journal.* 2 (1), 27-45.

Yontef, G. M. (1982). Gestalt therapy and its inheritance from Gestalt psychology. *Gestalt Therapy.* 4(1/2), 23-39.

Yontef, G. M. (1988). Assimilating diagnostic and psychoanalytic perspectives into Gestalt therapy. *Gestalt Journal.* 11 (1), 5-32.

Yontef, G. M. (1993). *Awareness, dialogue & process: Essays on Gestalt therapy*. New York: The Gestalt Journal Press, Inc.

Yontef, G. & Simkin, J. (1989). *Gestalt Therapy*. R. Corsini & D. Wedding (Eds). Current Psychotherapies, 4ᵗʰ edition. Itasca, IL:F.

E. Peacock Publishers.

Zeigarnik, B. (1927). Uber das behalten von erledigten und unerledigten handlungen. *Psychologische Forschung*. 9, 1-85.

Zinker, J. (1971). Dream work as theatre. Voices. 1 (2), summer. Zinker, J. (1977). Creative process in Gestalt therapy. New York:

Brunner/Mazel.

Zinker, J. (1990). Chapter 3. Harman R. L. (ed). Gestalt Therapy Discussions with the Masters, Charles C. Thomas Springfield: Illinois.

Zinker, J. C. (1994). In search of good form. A Gestalt institute of Cleveland publication. San Francisco. Jossey-Bass Publishers.

INDEX

A

action phase, 97

active techniques, 28

"aha" experience, 78, 246-47

anastropic expectations, 107

anger, 31, 44, 58, 62, 74, 83, 97, 103, 106, 115-17, 119, 122-23, 125, 139, 143, 163-64, 167, 170-71, 185-87, 190-91, 196, 199, 201- 5, 227, 230, 232, 272, 278, 285, 287, 294-95, 313, 318-21, 332- 34, 338, 340

anxiety, 27, 30-31, 41-42, 44, 58, 61-62, 83, 96-97, 99, 106-7, 135-36,161, 164, 167, 185, 195, 203, 213,262, 285, 287, 294, 296, 323

archetypes, 236, 345

assimilation, 92, 144, 157

authenticity, 27, 41

awareness, 15, 23, 29, 31, 45, 48-52,56, 63, 65, 69-85, 89, 91-97, 101,135, 166-67, 171, 192-93, 197,205, 209-10, 214, 233, 235, 243,246, 265, 268, 275-76, 278-81,290, 297, 299, 301, 304, 308-9,336, 338, 343-44, 348, 350, of environmental factors, 76 of feelings, 73 of internal experiences, 72 of the reconciliation field, 76 of sensations and behaviors, 73 of value judgments, 75 of wishes, 74

awareness phase, 95-96

awareness work, 80, 83-85, 209

B

bodily reactions, 14, 17, 59, 97, 272, 274-76, 280, 291

body armour, 28, 275-76

body boundaries, 135

body language, 271, 273, 275-76, 291-92, 303

body structure and posture, 17, 271, 289-91

C

catastrophic expectations, 107

cliché layer, 44

confluence, 16-17, 101, 138-39, 217-30, 232, 234-35, 324, 327-29

contact, pathways of, 130

The Gestalt approach is both a life philosophy and a therapy school. The Gestalt approach, with its humanistic point of view, gives the opportunity to the person to be aware of himself or herself and those around him or her to integrate both within himself or herself and with the world without judging or accusing, without feeling ashamed, scared, or worried, and to exist as fully grown in the way he or she really is. This book is written with two important goals in mind. One of the aims of the book is to introduce the Gestalt therapy approach and, while introducing it, to help the readers to be aware of their needs, wishes, the styles of contact they use in their relations, their unfinished businesses, their impasses, and their resistance to change. The second purpose of the book is to help those therapists in therapy training by presenting the theory and methods of the Gestalt approach with examples and thus contribute to the raising of their therapeutic knowledge and skill levels.

Prof. Dr. Ceylan Das is a clinical psychologist and psychotherapist. She has given lectures in the psychology departments of universities for years, and she also has her private practice. She works with individuals, couples, as well as with groups. She started her Gestalt therapy training with Metanoia, England, and continued with different Gestalt Institutes in Europe and the USA. She is the president of Turkish Gestalt Therapy Association and the editor of Contact: Gestalt Therapy Journal.

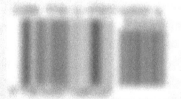

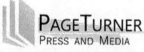

PAGETURNER
PRESS AND MEDIA

CPSIA information can be obtained
at www.ICGtesting.com
Printed in the USA
BVHW072037010321
601385BV00001B/61

9 781649 086327